Praise for the *Voices of* Book Series

"Pure inspiration."

Shape Magazine

"...provides answers to practically anyone wondering 'What now?' ...this worthy collection succeeds very well."

Publishers Weekly

"Hearing others' stories is the most substantial aspect of any support group... It's the universality of the emotions that links these essays and puts the human face on what can be a very scary disease. For all patient health collections."

Library Journal

Other Books by The Healing Project

Voices of Alcoholism
Voices of Alzheimer's
Voices of Autism
Voices of Caregiving
Voices of Breast Cancer
Voices of Lung Cancer

Voices of Multiple Sclerosis

The Healing Companion: Stories for Courage, Comfort and Strength

Edited by

The Healing Project

www.thehealingproject.org

"Voices Of" Series Book No. 7

LaChancepublishing

LACHANCE PUBLISHING • NEW YORK

www.lachancepublishing.com

Copyright © 2010 by LaChance Publishing LLC

ISBN 978-1-934184-08-0

Victor Starsia
Publisher

Richard Day Gore
Senior Editor

Juliann Garey
Associate Editor

Library of Congress Control Number: 2008927931

Publisher: LaChance Publishing LLC
              120 Bond Street
              Brooklyn, NY 11217
              www.lachancepublishing.com

Distributor: Independent Publishers Group
              814 North Franklin Street
              Chicago, IL 60610
              www.ipgbook.com

This book is available at special discounts for bulk purchases for sales promotions or premiums. Special editions, including personalized covers, excerpts of existing books, and corporate imprints, can be created in large quantities for special needs. For more information, write to LaChance Publishing, 120 Bond Street, New York, NY 11217 or email info@lachancepublishing.com.

Sometimes the journey from beginning to end is not always clear and straightforward. While work on *Voices Of* began just a short time ago, the seeds were planted long ago by beloved sources. This book is dedicated to Jennie, Larry and Denise, who in the face of all things good and bad gave courage and support in excess. But especially to Richard, who taught us by the way he lived his life that anything is possible given enough time, hard work and love.

Contents

Part I I Have MS

Part II   Now What?

Part III   Living with MS

The Healing Project
Debra LaChance

I wanted to ask the people around me, "Would you please raise
your hand if you feel as isolated as I do?" Walking the busy streets
of Manhattan on a beautiful sunny day, I was surrounded by people but I'd never felt so alone. Just minutes before, my doctors had
broken the news to me that I had a particularly aggressive form of
breast cancer.

Since moving to New York from a small town in Rhode Island, I'd
had my share of ups and downs but had always risen to the challenges that living and working in New York can bring. But on this
summer afternoon, I felt as if the world was suddenly rushing past
me while I seemed to be moving in slow motion. I was completely
alone.

After recovering from the initial shock, I found that one of the
first things I almost automatically began to look for, besides doctors, was a sense of connection. I needed to hear from other people who had gone through what I was experiencing, who truly
understood what it meant and who might be able to help. I was-
n't ready for a regular support group, and with surgery and treatment looming, I simply didn't have the time. But I am an avid
reader, and I assumed that finding the personal stories of those
who had gone through this ordeal before me would be relatively

easy. But there seemed to be a vacuum; almost nothing. Where were the real people to talk to? Where was the literature that wasn't just about the hardcore science of the disease, but about how to cope?

I knew there must be countless others out there who needed to tell their stories—and to hear the stories of others as well. My thoughts kept returning to that walk through Manhattan after I'd heard my diagnosis, and that feeling of terrible loneliness. As sympathetic as friends and loved ones could be, I felt that no one could truly understand this journey except someone who had made it before. I was convinced that getting and giving courage, comfort, and strength were as important as good medical care, and I became determined to help build a community for people like me who were undergoing the terribly isolating experience of dealing with a life-threatening or chronic disease.

Out of this resolve to build a sense of community, The Healing Project was born. The Healing Project's mission is to become a bridge across which people can make those all-important emotional connections. I began to develop The Healing Project as a place where people can contribute funds for research, time for connecting with others, and most of all, a place to share their stories. Since then, The Healing Project has been collecting stories by those touched by illness or diseases for books like this one: books that inspire and inform for the road ahead and impart a sense of community for those caught up in dealing with the moment. These books are meant to be a companion for patients, their friends, and families, an oasis where they can find strength in shared experiences. I don't want anyone to have to feel the way I did the day of my diagnosis when I was walking through the city alone and afraid. There's so much strength in others—you just have to find them.

When you are dealing with disease, you have to be ready to chart a new course, for the rest of your life, no matter what the outcome. And it helps to see that others are busy charting their own courses along with you. That's what these stories are all about. Reading these amazing contributions to the Voices Of series convinces me that I don't really have a uniquely remarkable story at all.

The truth is, everyone does.

―――――――――

Debra LaChance is the creator and founder of The Healing Project.

The Healing Project

Individuals diagnosed with life-threatening or chronic, debilitating illnesses face countless physical, emotional, social, spiritual, and financial challenges during their treatment and throughout their lives. The support of family members, friends, and the community at large is essential to their successful recovery and their quality of life, and access to accurate and current information about their illnesses enables patients and their caregivers to make informed decisions about treatment and post-treatment care. Founded in 2005 by Debra LaChance, *The Healing Project* is dedicated to promoting the health and well-being of these individuals, developing resources to enhance their quality of life, and supporting the family members and friends who care for them. For more information about *The Healing Project* and its programs, please visit our website at www.thehealingproject.org.

An Overview of
Multiple Sclerosis
John Richert, M.D.

Multiple sclerosis, or MS, is a chronic, often disabling disease of the *central nervous system (CNS)*, which is comprised of the brain, spinal cord, and optic nerves. MS is thought to be an autoimmune disease in which the immune system attacks the CNS. It was recognized as a distinct disease by the French neurologist Jean-Martin Charcot in 1868, but the earliest known description of a person with possible MS dates from 14th century Holland. There are currently at least 400,000 people with multiple sclerosis in the United States alone—with another 200 people diagnosed every week—and more than 2.1 million people are thought to have MS around the globe. Its progress, severity, and specific symptoms are unpredictable and can be very different from one person to another, which presents special challenges in the diagnosis and treatment of this widespread disease.

During an MS attack, inflammation occurs predominantly in the *white matter*, or nerve fibers of the central nervous system, in random patches called *plaques*. This process results in the destruction of *myelin*, the fatty covering that insulates nerve cell fibers, as well as the nerve fibers themselves. Myelin facilitates the smooth, high-speed transmission of electrochemical messages between the brain, the spinal cord, and the rest of the body. When myelin and the underlying nerve fiber are damaged, the transmission of messages may be slowed or blocked completely, leading to diminished or lost bodily function. The name "multiple sclerosis" signifies both the number (multiple) and the condition (sclerosis, from the Greek term for scarring or hardening) of the demyelinated areas in the central nervous system.

The Varieties of Multiple Sclerosis

Cases of multiple sclerosis typically fall into one of four "courses," each of which can range in severity from mild to severe. The disease course may appear very different from one person to another. Due to the many variables in how multiple sclerosis manifests itself, it can take some time for a physician to determine which course a person is experiencing. The disease courses are:

- **Relapsing-Remitting MS** is the most common form of the disease and approximately 85% of multiple sclerosis cases begin with this type of MS, which is characterized by clearly defined attacks of worsening neurologic function. These attacks, also known as relapses, flare-ups, or exacerbations, are followed by partial or complete recovery periods, known as *remissions*, during which there is no apparent disease progression.

- **Primary-Progressive MS** is characterized by slowly worsening neurologic function from the onset, without distinct relapses or remissions. The rate of progression may vary, with occasional plateaus and temporary minor improvements. Approximately 10% of people with multiple sclerosis have primary-progressive MS.

- **Secondary-Progressive MS.** In many patients, a secondary-progressive disease course follows an initial period of relapsing-remitting MS. In secondary-progressive MS, the disease worsens more steadily, with or without occasional flare-ups, remissions, or plateaus. Before disease-modifying medications became available, approximately 50% of people with relapsing-remitting MS developed secondary-progressive MS within 10 years of its onset.

- **Progressive-Relapsing MS** occurs in only about 5% of multiple sclerosis cases. People with this form of MS experience a steady worsening of the disease from the onset, with attacks of worsening neurologic function during the course of the illness. The disease continues to progress without remissions.

What Causes Multiple Sclerosis?

No one knows exactly what causes MS but we do understand much about the underlying processes involved. To understand what is happening when a person has MS, it's helpful to know a little about how the healthy immune system works. The immune system—a complex network of specialized cells and organs—defends the body against attacks by "foreign" invaders such as bacteria, viruses, fungi, and parasites. It does this by seeking out and destroying the interlopers as they enter the body. Substances capable of triggering an immune response against them are called *antigens*.

The immune system can recognize millions of distinctive foreign molecules and produces its own molecules and cells to counteract each of them. In order to have room for enough cells to match the millions of possible foreign invaders, the immune system stores just a few cells for each specific antigen. When an antigen appears, those few specifically matched cells are stimulated to multiply into a full-scale army. Later, to prevent this army from becoming too large, powerful mechanisms to suppress the immune response come into play.

T cells, so named because they are processed in the thymus gland, appear to play a particularly important role in MS. They travel widely and continuously throughout the body, patrolling for foreign invaders. In order to recognize and respond to each specific antigen, each T cell's surface carries special receptor molecules for particular antigens.

T cells contribute to the body's defenses in many ways. They can activate the body's defenses against foreign substances, and they can also turn off, or suppress, various immune system cells when their job is done. Another type of T cell can directly attack diseased or damaged body cells, and others release messenger chemicals called *cytokines* that stimulate other immune cells.

Since T cells can attack cells directly, they must be able to discriminate between "self" antigens (those of the body) and "nonself" antigens (belonging to foreign invaders). To prevent the immune system from attacking self antigens, T cells that are likely to react against them are usually eliminated before leaving the thymus, and the remaining self-reacting T cells are largely held in check by another class of T cells called "regulatory T cells." This enables the immune system to coexist peaceably with body tissues in a state of self-tolerance.

Recent research suggests that another type of immune cell, called the B cell, is also involved at some point during the course of MS. B cells produce antibodies which can attach to invaders—or tissues—and mark them for destruction by other immune forces. In MS, they may also play a role in "presenting" myelin fragments to T cells to stimulate attacks.

In autoimmune diseases such as MS, the peace between the immune system and the body is disrupted when the immune system seems to wrongly identify self as nonself and declares war on the part of the body (myelin, in the case of MS) that it no longer recognizes as self. Scientists believe a number of factors may contribute to the development of MS. Among them are:

Environmental Causes
Scientists are studying variations in geography, demographics, migration patterns, and infectious causes in an effort to under-

stand how environmental factors may impact the incidence of MS. Studies of migration patterns suggest that exposure to some environmental agent before or during puberty may predispose a person to develop MS later on, and it has also been shown that the farther one lives from earth's equator, the higher is the incidence of MS. It may be that naturally produced vitamin D from exposure to sunlight, which is thought to suppress the immune system, is a factor in the lower incidence of multiple sclerosis closer to the equator. Ongoing studies of MS clusters (discussed below) may eventually provide clues to other environmental factors such as industrial toxins, diet, or trace metal exposure that might cause or trigger MS.

Infectious Agents

It is possible that a virus or other infectious agent is behind MS, since some viruses are known to cause demyelination and nerve inflammation. More than a dozen viruses and bacteria, including measles, human herpes virus-6, Epstein-Barr, canine distemper, and Chlamydia pneumonia have been (or are being) studied to determine if they play some role in the development of MS, but thus far no infectious agent has been definitively identified as being responsible for triggering cases of MS.

Genetic Factors

Increasing scientific evidence suggests that genetics plays a role in determining a person's susceptibility to MS. If one person in a family has MS, that person's first-degree relatives—parents, children, and siblings—have a 30- to 50-fold higher chance of getting the disease than does the general population. For identical twins, the likelihood that the second twin may develop MS if the first twin has it is about 30 percent; for fraternal twins (who do not inherit identical gene pools), the likelihood is closer to that for non-twin siblings, or about 4 percent. The difference in concordance rates for identical vs. fraternal twins tells us that genetics plays a significant role, but the fact that the rate for the second identical twin developing MS is significantly less than 100 percent indicates that the disease is not entirely genetically controlled. As noted above, most of this non-genetic effect is likely due to an environmental exposure. Further evidence for a genetic role comes from populations that are, to varying degrees, resistant to developing MS despite living at geographic latitudes where MS is otherwise quite common. Romanis and Inuits appear to never get MS, and Native Americans, Japanese, and other Asian peoples have very low incidence rates.

Indications that multiple genes are involved in MS susceptibility come from studies of people with MS and family members. Of particular interest are the *human leukocyte antigen* (HLA) genes. HLAs are genetically determined proteins that influence the immune system. Certain HLA genes are found more frequently in people with MS compared to people without the disease. A number of other gene variants that are over-represented in the MS population have recently been identified and there is also growing evidence that different combinations of genes may relate to variations in disease severity and progression.

These and other studies strengthen the theory that MS is the result of a number of factors rather than a single gene or other agent. The development of MS is likely to be influenced by the interactions of a number of genes, each of which (individually) has only a modest effect. Additional studies, which are now underway, are needed to specifically pinpoint which genes are involved, determine their function, and learn how each gene's interactions with other genes and with the environment make an individual susceptible to MS.

Who Gets Multiple Sclerosis?

MS is two to three times more common in women than in men. MS can appear in young children and teens, though the majority of cases occur in adults between the ages of 20 and 50. It can appear in much older adults as well. As previously noted, the incidence of multiple sclerosis is higher in areas farther from the Equator.

Although MS occurs in most ethnic groups including African-Americans, Asians and Hispanics/Latinos, it is more common in Caucasians of northern European ancestry. Some ethnic groups, however, such as the Inuit, Aborigines and Maoris, report virtually no cases of MS, regardless of where they live. These variations, even within geographic areas with the same climate, suggest that geography, genes, and other factors interact in a complex way, underscoring the daunting nature of finding a cause and a cure for the disease. In addition, scientists are studying "MS clusters," in which a high number of cases of MS have occurred over a specific time period and in a certain geographical area, and this research may provide clues to environmental or genetic factors that might predispose to, cause, or trigger the disease.

The Symptoms of Multiple Sclerosis

Compounding the challenges that researchers face in studying multiple sclerosis is the fact that it can manifest itself as a wide variety of symptoms, which may appear in any combination or level of severity. Symptoms of MS include:

- Weakness, paralysis

- Walking, balance and coordination problems

- Numbness of the face, body, or extremities

- Vision problems, fatigue

- Pain

- Bladder dysfunction

- Bowel dysfunction

- Dizziness, vertigo

- Spasticity (feelings of stiffness and involuntary muscle spasms)

- Sexual dysfunction

- Cognitive difficulties

- Depression and other emotional changes

Many people with MS report abnormal sensations in their bodies, usually in their extremities, which they commonly refer to as "pins and needles" and "electric shocks." Less common symptoms of MS include speech disorders, problems swallowing, headache, seizures, hearing loss, tremor, problems with breathing, and itching.

Diagnosing Multiple Sclerosis

Arriving at a diagnosis of MS can be difficult and time-consuming because there is no single symptom, physical finding, or laboratory test that can, by itself, determine if a person has multiple sclerosis. To determine if a person meets the criteria for a diagnosis of MS (and to rule out other possible causes of the symptoms), doctors will carefully study the person's medical history, perform a neurologic exam, and order various tests, including those detailed below. It is generally accepted that, in order to make a diagnosis of MS, the physician must: find evidence of damage in at least two separate areas of the central nervous system; find evidence that the instances of damage occurred at least one month apart; *and* rule out all other possible diagnoses.

Medical History and Neurologic Examination

The physician obtains a thorough patient history to identify any past or present symptoms that might be, or might have been, caused by multiple sclerosis. Further clues about the cause of the patient's problems might be gathered from information on the birthplace, family history, and places the person has traveled. Motor function, balance, coordination, vision, and other sensory functions (for example, the ability to feel a pinprick or light touch) will be examined. Often strong evidence for a diagnosis of MS can be gathered from the person's medical history and neurologic exam. Other tests help confirm the diagnosis or provide additional evidence.

MRI

Magnetic resonance imaging (MRI) is the most effective imaging technology for detecting the presence of MS lesions (plaques) in the central nervous system. But MS can't be diagnosed just on the basis of MRIs, because some other diseases cause lesions that resemble those associated with MS. Similar spots can also appear in the brains of individuals with no active disease (for example, as a result of prior head trauma) and are also seen more commonly with advancing age. It should be noted that a normal MRI of the brain does not always rule out MS, and some 5% of those with MS do not initially have brain lesions detected on their MRIs. The longer a person's MRI does not show brain or spinal cord lesions, the more important it becomes to search for other possible diagnoses.

Visual Evoked Potentials (VEPs)

Evoked potentials (EPs), which represent the nervous system's electrical response to stimulation of specific pathways, such as visual, auditory and general sensory pathways, are recorded and analyzed for evidence of MS damage. Since damage to myelin (demyelination) causes slowing of response time, EPs can provide evidence that is not necessarily revealed by the neurologic exam. Visual evoked potentials are considered the most useful for helping to confirm a diagnosis of MS

Cerebrospinal Fluid Analysis

Analysis of the patient's cerebrospinal fluid can detect certain immune system proteins, particularly *oligoclonal bands* (bands of immunoglobulins, i.e. antibodies), which indicate an immune response within the central nervous system. Oligoclonal bands are found in the spinal fluid of about 90-95% of people with MS. However, they are also present in some other diseases, so they cannot be taken as absolute proof of MS.

Blood Tests

There is no definitive blood test for multiple sclerosis, but blood tests can help rule out other conditions that cause MS-like symptoms, such as Lyme disease, collagen-vascular diseases (e.g., systemic lupus erythematosus, rheumatoid arthritis), AIDS, syphilis, vitamin B_{12} deficiency, and certain rare hereditary disorders.

Treating Multiple Sclerosis

There is as yet no cure for MS. A small percentage of patients do well with no therapy at all but one cannot predict which people these will be. Although naturally occurring or spontaneous remissions complicate efforts to determine the therapeutic effects of experimental treatments, controlled clinical trials provide evidence that the FDA-approved disease-modifying medications are effective at reducing disease activity and disease progression, and appear to be especially beneficial if taken early in the course of the disease.

Treating the Symptoms of MS

As described above, MS can cause a wide variety of symptoms. Often, through a combination of physical therapy and drug treatment, the symptoms of MS can be eased. Spasticity can be addressed with a combination of medication, physical therapy, and mobility aids. Bladder problems are often treated with "anticholinergic" agents, such as oxybutin (Ditropan) and tolterodine (Detrol). Fatigue is often addressed by therapies that range from physical therapy to frequent naps, moderate exercise and drugs such as amantadine (Symmetrel) and modafinil (Provigil). MS-related "neurogenic" pain can be treated with a variety of medications, such as anti-seizure medications (e.g., carbamazepine [Tegretol]) and certain types of anti-depressants (e.g., amitriptyline [Elavil]). With regard to the latter, it is important to know, however, that the beneficial effects of drugs like amitriptyline seem not to be related to their anti-depressant effects and one does not need to be depressed in order to have his/her pain benefit from these anti-depressant medications.

Modifying the Disease

In the past, the principal medications that physicians used to treat MS were steroids possessing anti-inflammatory properties such as prednisone, methylprednisolone and prednisolone, and adrenocorticotropic hormone (better known as ACTH). These drugs can reduce the duration and severity of attacks in many patients. Because steroids can produce numerous adverse side effects (hypertension, diabetes, bone loss and mood changes, among others), they are not recommended for long-term use at high dosage frequencies. There is, however, limited evidence suggesting that infrequent pulses of steroids (e.g, monthly) may have some long term benefit on disease activity.

Since 1993, six drugs have been approved by the Food and Drug Administration for use in reducing the activity of the disease in many patients. While they are not cures for MS, they have been shown to provide significant long-term benefit for people with relapsing forms of MS. Three such drugs, Avonex, Betaseron, and Rebif, known as *beta interferons*, have the capacity to both modulate the immune system and interfere with the behavior of viruses in the body. They reduce the number of exacerbations and also slow the progression of physical disability. When attacks do occur, they tend to be shorter and less severe. In addition, MRI scans suggest that beta interferon can decrease myelin destruction.

Potential side effects of interferons include fever, chills, sweating, muscle aches, fatigue, depression, and injection site reactions.

Glatiramer acetate (Copaxone) is a synthetic compound that is thought to stimulate the T cells in the body's immune system to change from harmful, pro-inflammatory agents to more beneficial, anti-inflammatory agents that work to reduce inflammation at lesion sites in the central nervous system. It, too, has been approved for people with relapsing MS.

Another approved treatment for MS is natalizumab (Tysabri) a *monoclonal antibody* (a laboratory-produced antibody) that is designed to hamper the movement of immune cells within the body. In 2006, the FDA approved the sale of the drug for MS under strict treatment guidelines involving infusion centers where patients can be monitored by specially trained physicians. With natalizumab, there appears to be an approximately one-in-one-thousand risk of developing a severe viral infection of the nervous system called progressive multifocal leukoencephalopathy (PML).

Finally, the immunosuppressant drug mitoxantrone (Novantrone), has been approved by the FDA for the treatment of worsening MS. It has been used to reduce the frequency of relapses in patients with secondary-progressive MS, progressive-relapsing MS or worsening relapsing-remitting MS. Both mitoxantrone and natalizumab are generally reserved for use in patients who have had sub-optimal responses to the interferons and/or glatiramer acetate.

Other Treatments for MS

Plasma exchange, or *plasmapheresis*, is a procedure by which blood is removed from the patient and the plasma is separated from other blood substances and discarded. Plasma contains antibodies and other immunologically active products. The remaining components of blood are then transfused back into the patient. Because its worth as a treatment for MS has not yet been proven, this procedure is still largely experimental. Nevertheless, there are instances when MS physicians feel that it is worth trying, usually when a patient has been refractory to other more standard treatments.

Bone marrow transplantation is an experimental procedure for MS that is performed in hopes of "rebooting" the immune system. Certain bone marrow cells from the individual are stored, then re-infused after the patient undergoes drug therapy (and sometimes radiation therapy) to kill their immune cells. The long-term effectiveness of this procedure is not yet known, and it carries potentially severe risks, including death.

Bee venom injections have been espoused in some quarters in attempts to treat MS. There is no definitive evidence that it can produce lasting benefit, and it carries the risk of potentially severe side effects, particularly related to allergic reactions, including anaphylaxis.

Because the transmission of electrochemical messages within the central nervous system is disrupted in MS, medications to improve the conduction of nerve impulses are being investigated. Since blocking certain channels through which potassium moves improves conduction of the nerve impulse (improving the velocity of the electrical impulse), drugs that block these potassium channels have been developed in order to improve symptoms of MS. In several experimental trials, derivatives of a drug called aminopyridine temporarily improved MS symptoms, particularly walking ability. This drug has been formulated into a time-release capsule called Fampridine, which the FDA is currently reviewing. A decision about the drug's approval is expected in late 2009.

As growing insights into the workings of the immune system provide new knowledge about the function of *cytokines*, the powerful chemicals produced by T cells, the possibility of using them to manipulate the immune system becomes more attractive. Scientists are studying a variety of substances that may block harmful cytokines, such as those involved in inflammation, or that encourage the production of protective cytokines.

Many studies focus on strategies to reverse the damage to myelin and *oligodendrocytes* (the cells that make and maintain myelin in the central nervous system), both of which are destroyed during MS attacks. Scientists now know that oligodendrocytes are capable of proliferating and forming new myelin after an attack, though they become less able to do this as the disease progresses. Therefore, there is a great deal of interest in agents or cell therapies that may stimulate this reaction. The concept of "neuroprotection" is also on the forefront of MS research: finding agents that may actually protect brain and spinal cord tissues from damage seems feasible. Drugs such as lamotrigine, an anti-convulsant, and riluzole, which is approved for ALS, are currently being tested.

Over the years, many people have tried to implicate diet as a cause of, or treatment for, MS. Some physicians have advocated a diet low in saturated fats; others have suggested increasing the patient's intake of linoleic acid, a polyunsaturated fat, via supplements of sunflower seed, safflower, or evening primrose oils. Other proposed dietary "remedies" include megavitamin therapy, including increased intake of vitamins B_{12} or C; various liquid diets; and sucrose-or gluten-free diets. To date, clinical studies have not been able to confirm benefits from dietary changes. In the absence of any evidence that diet therapy is effective, patients are best advised to eat a balanced, low-fat, high fiber diet that is healthy from many standpoints.

Recent Advances in Multiple Sclerosis Research

Many advances, on several fronts, have been made in treating and understanding MS. Each advance interacts with the others, adding greater depth and meaning to each new discovery.

Over the last decade, our knowledge about how the immune system works has grown at an amazing rate. Major gains have been made in recognizing and defining the role of this system in the development of MS lesions, giving scientists the ability to devise ways to alter the immune response. Such work is expected to yield a variety of new potential therapies. New tools such as MRI have redefined the natural history of MS and are proving invaluable in monitoring disease activity. Scientists are now able to visualize and follow the development of MS lesions in the brain and spinal cord using MRI. This ability is a tremendous aid in the assessment of new therapies and can speed the process of evaluating new treatments.

Other tools have been developed that make the painstaking work of discovering the disease's genetic secrets possible. Such studies have strengthened scientists' conviction that MS is a disease with many genetic components, none of which is dominant. Immune system-related genetic factors that predispose an individual to the development of MS have been identified, and some of these are pointing toward new potential therapeutic targets, some of which are already the subject of early stage clinical trials.

A growing number of therapies are now available that effectively treat the underlying course of MS, and some are available that treat MS symptoms. In addition, there are a number of treatments under investigation, some of them now oral rather than injected or infused, that may curtail attacks or improve function of demyelinated nerve fibers. The first two oral disease modifying therapies, cladribine and fingolimod, are expected to be submitted to the FDA for review before the close of 2009. The first symptom management oral therapy to improve walking ability, Fampridine, has already been submitted to the FDA for review. Over a dozen clinical studies testing potential therapies are in late stage trials moving through the MS pipeline, and additional new treatments, including therapies aimed at repairing MS damage, are being devised and tested in animal models.

Multiple Sclerosis and the Future

Although more cases of MS are being reported than in the past, there is no clear evidence that the disease is generally on the increase. Rather, the phenomenon most likely stems from increased awareness of MS, improved medical care, and advances in the tools and strategies used to reach a diagnosis. Nevertheless, there is evidence of increased MS incidence in several restricted population regions, such as Sardinia and Kuwait. There is currently an effort to secure funding for a new federally sponsored incidence and prevalence study in the U.S., which would answer questions about changing patterns of MS in this country.

At present there is no cure for multiple sclerosis, but to the countless scientists, physicians and researchers who are bringing us closer to understanding the cause of MS, it is not "incurable." They are working, together and separately, on new medications and therapies, breaking ground to discover new ways in which multiple sclerosis can be treated and, ultimately, cured and prevented. To be certain, the role of genetic risk factors, and how they can be modified, must be more clearly defined. Environmental triggers, such as viruses or toxins, need to be investigated further. The specific cellular and subcellular targets of immune attack in the brain and spinal cord, and the subsets of immune cells involved in that attack, need to be identified. Knowledge of these aspects of the disease will enable scientists to develop new, more specific methods for halting—or reversing and repairing—the destruction of myelin and nerve fibers. But the field of MS research is ever-growing, and progress is being made. Though it is impossible to say definitively when the breakthroughs of cure and prevention will occur, they are coming.

John Richert, M.D., is the Executive Vice President of Research & Clinical Programs for the National Multiple Sclerosis Society. He heads the world's leading MS biomedical, clinical and healthcare policy research initiatives and oversees the Society's extensive professional information and education programs.

Dr. Richert earned his medical degree from the University of Rochester Medical School. He completed his residency in Neurology at the Mayo

Clinic, and then pursued his interest in myelin and immunology by accepting a postdoctoral fellowship from the National MS Society to work at the National Institutes of Health. He joined the faculty of Georgetown University in 1980, where he served as Professor and Chair of the Department of Microbiology and Immunology, Professor of Neurology, and Director of the Georgetown MS Research Center. Dr, Richert has authored and co-authored over 100 journal articles and many other publications, and was a long-time volunteer for the National MS Society before joining the Society's staff in 2005.

Under his leadership, the Society has launched bold new strategic efforts to increase its role as a driving force of MS research, including funding large-scale, breakthrough projects like an international effort to map the genome of MS, the first large-scale clinical trial of estriol in women with MS, and the Society's Fast Forward drug development initiative. Under his guidance, the Society also convened a major stem cell research summit and launched task forces on the epidemiology of MS, long term care issues, and the use of cannabis. Dr. Richert is currently leading the development of a roadmap for future MS research directions.

Angels Fly

Teri Garr

Last summer, my darling daughter Molly and I went to the Hollywood Bowl for the Fourth of July Spectacular with my friend Heidi and her 13 year-old daughter, Haley. As usual, I over-packed: picnic basket, cooler, and a bunch of crap we really didn't need. It was eighty-five degrees, and the hike to our seats was way longer than we'd imagined. Soon I was limping a little and, well, the show must go on, so I was afraid my difficulty was going to make us late.

But lo, yonder galloped Prince Charming, riding one of those drive-around-the-parking-lot electric golf carts. I stuck out my thumb in the universal gesture of Dude, I need a ride. My Prince Charming (actually an unemployed actor/groundskeeper) saw this damsel in distress as he approached on his charger.

"I'm not going your way."

And he zoomed past us. I wasn't being lazy or looking for sympathy. I needed a ride. How was he to know I have MS, and that something as ordinary as a stroll with a picnic basket can be very challenging, to say the least.

Challenge indeed: not long after my knight and his electric steed left us to our devices, this damsel in distress fell over, right on her butt, in front of all those concertgoers. I fall regularly, so it isn't really a big deal, even though Hollywood can be pretty merciless to people with—I hate the word—disabilities. I have plenty of experience with that, just like I have plenty of experience with multiple sclerosis.

Of course, much of my experience with MS came before I even knew I had it.

For years, I'd experienced a host of symptoms: tingling, weakness, numbness (I mean *numbness*) in my right leg, and enough fatigue to make me sleep twelve hours a night. This is never any good, but it's really not good when you work in Hollywood. The movie business doesn't just run on the perception of glamour and care-free living, it runs on (gasp, I know this is a huge surprise) money. Making movies is expensive, and often, before a performer is signed to work in a film, he or she must have a medical examination to satisfy the production's astronomically expensive insurers he or she is up for the task. I was more than happy for these cursory inspections to reveal nothing of the symptoms I'd been having for years and—surprise number two—I didn't bother to mention them. I had put many years of hard work into getting to that magical point in my career trajectory that all performers dream of: the point where the phone rings constantly with offers of continued employment.

Over the years, I'd seen a lot of doctors. Hearing tests. Vision tests. Electric wires to see if my hand jerked properly. A spinal tap. MS had come up in some conversations, but I always ended up "fine." Fine? Let me tell you what's not fine: having a guy on the film crew ask you, "Why do you walk like you have a stick up your butt?" How's that for glamour? But the truth is, sometimes I did because of the numbness in my leg.

Doctor after doctor, tests showed nothing. "You might have MS," offered one sage, "you might not." Thanks. Another thought the answer might be to read a book about meditation. Yeah, I'll relax, access my inner Gandhi and think away the pins and needles. The symptoms weren't constant though, and I spent half my time forgetting there was anything wrong with me, and the other half being fed up with the manifestations of my mystery ailment.

Then, in 1989, I went to a doctor in Boston who was a specialist in MS. I mentioned this appointment to the wrong "friend." She promptly carried this insider information to another "friend," and before long it was as if they had set up a *Terri Garr Has MS* phone line. I woke up one morning, ran a couple of miles at the gym, got home, drank a glass of orange juice, and suddenly I was in Condolence Central. Even people I'd seen only days or months before seemed to think I'd suddenly been forever confined to a wheelchair. Dealing with that was bad enough, but then my work opportunities suddenly fell off a cliff. The press was hungry to know more, but as for offers for work, my phone stopped ringing.

At first I was outraged. Whatever had been going on in my body had been doing so for years, and it had never gotten in the way of my work. Now, here I was, felled by a rumor! If I'd had an office job, I could have sued. Ironically enough, not too long after that I had another round of detailed tests, including an MRI. No MS. What I didn't know then was that multiple sclerosis is very, very sneaky. I like to say MS is to disease what Enron is to accounting. No rules. It's a big fat cheater. Luckily, it didn't cheat me out of my career. Not quite, anyway, but it was hard going from being a busy Oscar nominee to having to reassure producers and directors that I could do my job.

By the late 90s, I had done my best to learn to ignore what MS was or wasn't doing to my body, or what the legions of doctors could or couldn't tell me. Then, finally, I made an appointment that would change my life, with Dr. Leslie Weiner, Chairman and Professor of Neurology at the U.S.C. School of Medicine. Finally, Dr. Weiner was the first to say, "You probably have MS," and he immediately suggested some drug therapies. I wondered why, after all this time and all these doctors, I wasn't already on one.

People always ask, "What was it like when you got your diagnosis? Was it shocking? Did you cry?" All I say is no. After all I had gone through to get a diagnosis—any diagnosis—this news was anything but traumatic. In fact, it was quite a relief. After twenty years (that's twenty, 20) of maybes, I finally had something concrete to work with. I know this news can be devastating for some people, but Dr. Weiner said, "The Chinese word for crisis contains two characters, one meaning danger and the other meaning opportunity." It meant I had a 50-50 chance. He put me on one of the disease modifying therapies, Rebif, and I'm sure it has helped because I feel better and have fewer lesions on my MRI's. Wow. All it took was an actual diagnosis.

I'd done the danger part; now MS brought opportunity. David Lander (best known for playing "Squiggy" on *Laverne and Shirley*), who had been diagnosed with MS in 1984 but didn't go public until 1999, suggested I take a public stance about my MS. He said it could make others feel better. I was a bit hesitant at first, but he turned out to be so right. I became an Ambassador in the MS movement working for MS LifeLines, an educational and support service, and volunteering with the National Multiple Sclerosis Society.

I'll never forget the first time I gave a speech to an MS crowd. I didn't know what to expect from this first talk. Would I feel exposed and vulnerable? No; in fact it felt nothing like that at all. I stood at the podium and looked out at the men and women from all walks of life, some in wheelchairs, some sporting canes. This crowd offered a connection that most performers could barely dream of. They all shared something very personal with me: they all had their own MS stories to tell, either about themselves or about a loved one. These people knew what I'd been through. All the crazy things that had gone on with my body, that at times had made me feel so alone, were no longer so singular to me. There was a real, tangible camaraderie in this group. We were, and are, in it together.

Connecting with others and helping them through humor has been a wonderful experience. For people going through the fear and uncertainty of seeking a diagnosis (and getting one), it may seem hard to believe that there can be so much laughter in the MS community. But it's true, and we can all laugh together about such things as tripping on the corners of our rugs. I'm amazed wherever I go by the courage and good humor of the people I meet. One T-shirt worn by a man in a wheelchair made quite an impression: I'M NOT HANDICAPPED. I'M JUST TIRED. I've found that when we approach our MS without self-pity, those around us don't pity us, either. There's a saying I once heard: Angels fly because they take themselves lightly. In my quest for ways to deal with my illness, those words struck just the right chord. I've learned that my words and jokes can help others who are struggling to keep their spirits dancing while their bodies are dancing to another song entirely.

Meeting so many others with MS has helped me realize I am not defined by this disease, but by what's inside of me. I don't do well when I'm forced to look at the dark side; does anyone, really? So I prioritize keeping my chin up, like I prioritize my daily tasks. I used to be able to do fifty things in a day (by that I mean eight), and now I do four (and by that I mean one.) As long as that one thing isn't twisting off a childproof bottle cap or climbing 800 stairs, I'm fine. Come to think of it, I always had a hard time with childproof bottle caps, anyway.

But back to the Hollywood Bowl. Let me tell you, hiking to your seat in 85-degree heat, with a picnic basket, cooler, and a bunch of crap you don't need, can be a lot worse than climbing 800 stairs. So there I was, an MS Ambassador on my butt as concert-goers walked by. Haley and Molly laughed, and my friend Heidi and I joined them. An usher saw us and offered to send someone to help. We waited and waited, but nobody came and the show was about to start. We got me to my feet, and, determined not to give up, I started up the road again, our picnic supplies getting heavier with every difficult step. All of a sudden, Molly and Haley started chanting:

"I think I can, I think I can. I know I can, I know I can..."

My daughter bounced as she sang, full of energy, and I felt a surge of strength. All four of us sang along as we became the little engines that could.

I guess you could say that applies to the many wonderful people I meet as I travel around speaking about MS. We're not just little engines that could. We're little engines that *can*.

Teri Garr is one of America's best-loved comedic actresses, with film credits including *Young Frankenstein*, *Close Encounters of the Third Kind*, and *Mr. Mom*, and she garnered an Academy Award nomination for her supporting role in *Tootsie*. While continuing her acting career, she has embraced her role as National Ambassador for the National Multiple Sclerosis Society, touching thousands of people around the MS world with her humor and insight.

Acknowledgments

This book would not have been possible without the selfless dedication of many people giving freely of their valuable time and expertise. We'd particularly like to thank Arney Rosenblat and Dr. John R. Richert of the National Multiple Sclerosis Society for lending their extraordinary expertise and unflagging support; Ms. Teri Garr for her dedication to raising awareness of multiple sclerosis; and the many people who contributed their stories to us, for their courage, their generosity and their humanity.

Part I
I Have MS

Francis Scott Key
David Scaffidi

I was nervous, even scared. I had never really spent much time in a hospital before. Yet there I was, in Baltimore's Francis Scott Key Hospital. I was there because I'd had various problems. Odd problems, difficult to explain. The first of these had occurred the year before: I couldn't walk or use my hands, my speech slurred and a bout of vomiting went on, almost continuously, for three weeks. It was so unreal to me, only nineteen and having just begun university in New York. After those symptoms ended, I simply forgot about them. Forgetting them was easy at the time: three doctors each offered a different diagnosis that included severe vertigo, Ménière's disease, and something else equally vague. I didn't have an MRI, maybe because in 1988 MRIs were still prohibitively expensive.

But the symptoms did return. Now, in my Baltimore hospital room, I was placed across from a fidgety, slightly cantankerous older man. He confided that he was there because he had Parkinson's disease. He appeared optimistic and, cracking a wry smile, said he was taking an experimental medication. I admired his frank, detached, determined resolve. I'd never met someone in an experimental medical program, and imagined how difficult it would be to go through something like that.

Cowering in my bed, I dreaded the mysterious diagnostics that lay ahead: tests with odd names like VEP, MRI, EKG, EEG. The nurse came, but I only vaguely registered her presence. I was nauseous. I was scared. But she finally got my attention. She was roughly my age. Her big, beautiful blue eyes are what I remember most from that day. The day of my diagnosis.

> "I was about to get a diagnosis that would—that will—burden me for the rest of my life."

The pretty nurse gave me a small, silvery balloon that read, "Get well". I didn't know where she got it. I didn't care. I was sweating and cold. She was sweet. I was sick. She was pretty. I was scared. She kept coming back, and back, poking her head past the partition to see me. I tried to focus on her eyes to distract me from my fears.

I didn't know it then, but my fears would come true. I was about to get a diagnosis that would—that will—burden me for the rest of my life.

David Scaffidi lived in Maryland when diagnosed with relapsing-remitting MS. He was referred to the National Institutes of Health and treated there for over ten years. He left a doctoral program in psychology and neuroscience to write about MS and the coping strategies he learned. He's never lost hope, confident a cure will be found.

Living Triumphantly

Jodene Kersten

My mom's multiple sclerosis has become such a part of our lives that I sometimes forget that she has not always had it. She was diagnosed with the disease at 18 and yet, despite her doctors' misgivings, had two children in her mid-twenties. For the next 36 years she continued to selectively follow her physicians' orders to the frustration and amazement of specialists, neurologists, and her own family. At 62 she has slowed down a bit, but does not blame the change of pace on MS. The disease is now at the secondary progressive stage, which she bluntly calls "the end stage." She recently retired after 21 years as a full time neonatal intensive care nurse and occasionally, will still joke about her health, saying, "Denial for the past twenty-five years has worked great!" MS may be part of her life, but it has never defined her.

Mom was born at a Japanese-American relocation camp in Heart Mountain, Wyoming during World War II. Despite having American citizenship, my grandparents and extended family spent four years in the camp, accepting their circumstances and making the best of inhumane conditions. In 1946, after the end of the war, a generous Mormon family in Ogden, Utah sponsored our family out of the camp and my grandfather sharecropped on the family's land for a year to make enough money to return to their own farm in Arroyo Grande, California. After five years in Arroyo Grande, my grandfather left farming for a better life and moved his family of five to Los Angeles.

Mom describes herself as "the typical second child" who was constantly on the move and constantly in trouble. My grandmother calls her "the most challenging of all four girls" and my mom still recalls my grandfather often repeating, "I know you can do better" to mediocre reports cards. During junior high school our family moved to the San Gabriel Valley where the kids were the only Japanese-Americans in the school. Yet Mom never saw herself as different from the other students. Like other Japanese-Americans after the war, my grandparents encouraged their children to view themselves as Americans. Mom's attitude continued into high school, where she was a member of the Red Cross Club and Drill Team, never missed a dance or social function, and enjoyed being in the popular clique. She still jokes with my father about being her high school's Prom Queen.

In February 1963, during the middle of her freshman year at California State University at Los Angeles, Mom began to suffer physical exhaustion. She remained in college and was active in her sorority and as a Song Leader, but began sleeping up to 18 hours a day and maintaining her social commitments became a challenge. She began to lose her sense of balance, suffered from dizziness and experienced tingling and numbness in her left hand and foot. She soon lost hearing in both ears and vision in her left eye. Since her family physician could not find a cause to her illness, my grandmother took her to my great-grandmother's Japanese doctor in Los Angeles. Mom recalls that at that time, Magnetic Resonance Imaging (MRI) was not available so the physician, based on her symptoms, worked through a process of elimination and eventually provided an accurate diagnosis. She was then referred to a doctor at Huntington Memorial Hospital in Pasadena who was actively researching MS. Instead of medication, he prescribed a program of substantial rest and a diet of limited dairy products and no red meat, since he suspected that chemicals in the meat adversely interacted with nerve cells. Since then, she has followed the diet religiously and believes it has kept her healthy and active.

Mom remained in college until her junior year then decided to pursue nursing. She completed medical assistant school then worked in doctors' offices for three years while still living in Los Angeles. During this time, her high school sweetheart proposed. He had been by her side during the initial diagnosis and was aware of how MS affected her. She recalls "giving him an out" by telling him he didn't have to marry her, because she didn't know how severe the disease would become. Her greatest fear, then and now, is the loss of independence and reliance on a wheelchair. She didn't want him to feel responsible for her health care, but like my mom, he didn't allow MS to make his decisions and they married in 1966.

In 1970, my parents moved from Los Angeles to San Diego, where my father began his career as a school teacher, my sister was born and my mom opened a home daycare so she could be home with me and my sister. For six years she managed the daycare alone, opening the front door at 6 o'clock in the morning and sending home the last child at 6 o'clock at night. Once I began kindergarten in 1976, my mom returned to nursing school. At the end of her program she experienced her first relapse. After spending too much time in the sun, she became overheated and experienced weakness, exhaustion and a tingling in her extremities. While in the hospital, her physician treated the relapse with steroids but discovered she was part of the 1% of the population that suffers from a severe reaction to steroid treatment. She lost the use of her legs. After eight weeks of oral steroids she eventually recovered. Since the initial relapse, she has had four more hospital stays along with intense steroid treatment.

In 2002 while working twelve hour shifts as a fulltime NICU nurse, her health began to deteriorate. She felt increasingly exhausted. In late 2003, she underwent back surgery to remove a vertebrae crushed by the effects of severe osteoporosis. She assumed that after a few months she would return to work and resume her hectic schedule; however, due to trauma suffered to her nerves in her back her left leg became flaccid. After several months of being unable to work, her employer required her to take a medical retirement. Mom was devastated. She was only 59 and loved going to work. She felt that her identity was being taken away. She cried for several months as she dealt with the medical trauma, forced retirement and the search for a new identity. For an individual as strong and independent as Mom, this series of events was completely demoralizing.

After her retirement she experienced several minor MS relapses which were treated with steroids. She also completed three months of physical therapy for her back. As her MS progressed, she tried Novantrone, which was intended to last for two years; yet after one year, her doctor noticed little progress. She now uses a cane to steady her walk and an orthotic on her left leg for severe foot drop.

Her doctor has identified plaques on her spine, where demyelination has occurred. He is not certain if the plaques are reversible and suggests that steroid treatment will alleviate the severe inflammation. If that's the case, she might regain some leg movement. She also visits a licensed Asian medicine doctor and M.D. who has focused on improving her circulation. This approach has relieved some of her exhaustion and increased her energy level. The concern shared by Mom and her doctor is the over-stimulation of her immune system, which can cause a relapse. Maintaining her health requires ample rest, a strict diet, and a delicate balance of both western and eastern medicine. She no longer sits on the floor like she used to, but continues to maintain care of the inside of her home and do as much as she can.

When Mom and I sat on my couch to write her story, she regretted the ways MS has impacted our lives. I watched my two year-old sitting on her lap, content to play with her fingers and listen to the conversation. As she reflected on the past, I tried to identify personal or family adjustments made because of the disease, but it was impossible. MS is simply part of our lives. Mom finally mentioned how MS kept us from enjoying activities that other families did—like going on hot vacations. As she finished her sentence, we laughed because it sounded ridiculous. Since Mom cannot tolerate heat, I grew up in beautiful San Diego and doctors wrote Mom prescriptions for swimming pools. I thought I was the luckiest kid alive.

There are moments when I marvel at how she defies the odds. When we hear about celebrities or friends diagnosed with MS and their rapid decline, I have to remind myself of how devastating this disease can be. Mom has managed to control her MS. It does not define her. She believes that diet, rest and living in a cool, temperate environment have kept her well. We also know that my dad's support and fierce devotion have made a world of difference. He says "no" to favors asked by friends and family, and this has kept her healthy. Perhaps it's her spirit and will to prove others wrong, such as a cousin who recently said, "We didn't think you'd live to see 60!" For many, this comment could be devastating. For our family, it's a reminder of how my mom has successfully managed this disease.

> "I grew up in beautiful San Diego and doctors wrote Mom prescriptions for swimming pools. I thought I was the luckiest kid alive."

Recently she hinted at the possibility of great- grandkids. I joked that my oldest son, who is now six, won't be having children until his late 30s which would put her around 100. She reminded me that our family members live a long time. My great grandmother lived to 94 and my grandmother is independent at age 88, so it's not out of the question. We rarely mention MS because up to this point, it hasn't controlled her life. We remind the grandkids not to knock over grandma as they race through the house, but I'm guessing this is common in many households. We cannot know how MS will continue to impact her and the ones who love her. Lately, Mom has become increasingly frustrated with the disease, but she continues to live strong. She is living for her husband, her children, her mother and friends. She is living for her grandchildren. Most importantly, after 44 years of managing MS, she continues to live triumphantly.

Jodene Kersten is an assistant professor in Education at California State Polytechnic University Pomona. She lives with her spouse and two goofy boys in Agoura Hills, California. She spends most of her time behind a computer, with her nose in a book or playing at Malibu Beach with her family.

Living (and Sometimes Laughing) with Multiple Sclerosis
Melissa Scholes Young

At six petite pounds my daughter simply slipped softly into the world. I wept happy tears and healed, Isabelle nursed noisily and sprouted, and my husband Joe crashed into us both. For the first few days following Isabelle's birth, we struggled to be the perfect Pampers commercial: A happy couple laughs as they powder their baby's precious parts and change diapers…. They embrace in the dark while peering over the white, latticed crib as their angelic newborn snoozes…. The smiling lovers casually stroll together down the tulip-lined sidewalks and share their baby's cherubic slobber with neighbors.

But amidst the joy and stress, my devoted partner began slipping away. At first, Joe just seemed tired. Who isn't exhausted with a newborn and midnight nursings and crack-of-dawn diaperings? Our worries over money were also endless. Between my husband's measly graduate school stipend and my public school teaching paycheck, we quickly plunged into poverty.

As Isabelle and I bonded, Joe seemed to become more removed. Then he reported dizziness and nausea. Soon he didn't trust himself to hold the baby. And then one day my healthy, strong husband collapsed at a bathroom sink and lost all muscle control. He couldn't stand or even pull himself into a sitting position, and he wavered near unconsciousness. With the panicked help of neighbors we folded Joe into the car, strapped Isabelle into her seat and rushed to the emergency room.

Many perplexed doctors later, Joe was loaded into a wheelchair and sent home with drugs to wait for more tests. The best the doctors could tell us was that he had a severe case of labyrinthitis, a fancy word for ear infection, due to a head trauma. During the course of the doctor's interrogations, it was revealed that my husband had knocked himself silly several weeks before by banging his precious brain on an exposed pipe in our basement while playing indoor fetch with our overzealous puppy.

We laughed nervously over the diagnosis and tried to pretend the explanation was really that simple. I tucked us all into bed to recuperate. Joe drifted in and out of consciousness and proclaimed the holiness of the wondrous drugs while I drifted towards insanity with an infant who refused to sleep and a husband who did nothing but sleep.

> "When you are young and fearless you just can't imagine anything proving you otherwise."

Joe didn't get better. His nausea worsened and he began vomiting. The doctors kept telling us that he simply needed more rest and less stress. The wheelchair that had moved him easily around the hospital was absent in our three story home; neither of us could find the courage to broach the subject of its potential necessity. I locked myself in the bathroom one day for a good cry and realized that the façade was breaking down. Between sobs I called Joe's mother and asked her to fly up and sprinkle around some of her famous fairy dust. Joe and I had passed on the doctor's perplexing diagnosis, but we hadn't fully shared his condition with our family. I think we were in new baby bliss and denial ourselves. When you are young and fearless you just can't imagine anything proving you otherwise.

With the help of Joe's mother, we returned to the hospital with our now 10 day-old baby for another round of MRIs. The doctors were now convinced that something was terribly wrong with my otherwise healthy husband. Yet no one was ready to give us a verdict, and we were simply not prepared to process anything else. Again, the doctors sent us home to worry, to wait, to medicate. Joe began walking again, but he had lost a lot of weight and was now very weak. He still didn't trust himself to hold Isabelle, and he cried with shame once when he stumbled and sent our baby tucked in her car seat flying across the floor. Luckily, she was okay.

Joe was finally diagnosed with multiple sclerosis when our newborn was two months and two days old. At the most joyous time of our lives, the world came crashing down as if struck by a wrecking ball. At first, Joe sank into an unbearable and exhausting depression, and my carefree, spontaneous husband became a serious, melancholy old man overnight. His mood slowly bounced back with his health, but the trip was rattled with many late night doubts and what-if conversations I had never imagined when I said "I do." There were endless doctor's visits coupled with endless doctor's bills. Our baby, though, was our light and laughter through our adjustment to the daily demands of the diagnosis. We both turned our attention towards her amazing and happy simplicity. In her new discoveries about the world Joe and I slowly learned to take things more day-to-day.

For the past three years, Joe has visited a plethora of doctors, herbalists, and gurus. We've taken an eclectic approach to managing the disease and it mostly works for us. Joe even manages a startling sense of humor. He sings out to call me to the multiple daily injections, "Honey, it's time to stick needles in my bum!"

There are days, though, when Joe is simply not available. He's too exhausted to move, his thoughts are scrambled, and he scrunches up his face, struggling to answer simple questions. Those are the days when I feel really alone and terrified. Those are the days when there is little laughter. Joe, Isabelle and I somehow muddle through the lows, clinging to each other. So far our love is stronger than the prognosis. When we emerge on the other side of an attack, Joe smiles again and jokes, "See, honey, that wasn't so bad."

Melissa Scholes Young grew up in Hannibal, Missouri. When she is not finger painting with her daughter Isabelle, she teaches English and Creative Writing at Lincoln High School. Her publication credits include *Family Forum Magazine, A Cup of Comfort for Teachers, Literary Mama, The Front Porch Magazine,* and *The Tallahassee Democra*

On Satan, Signs, and Rabbi Akiva

Staci Bernard-Roth

"You don't have MS," said the neurologist, whom I was meeting for the first time. My family physician had called him a genius but warned me that he had no bedside manner. He was right about the bedside manner part.

Contrary to the neurologist's proclamation, I had been diagnosed with MS 11 years before. I had dutifully started seeing an MS specialist, but when he stopped taking my insurance and the MS seemed to go into remission, I didn't bother finding someone new—a big mistake. Now here I was with two numb feet and a doctor who apparently hadn't bothered to look at the medical records I braved the rain to drop off the day before.

"Um … I'm pretty sure I have it. Did you see? I was diagnosed by one of the best doctors in the country. She was sure I have it."

"You don't have it."

"Then why are my feet numb?"

"That's what we're trying to find out."

This new doctor—I'll call him "Satan"—ordered a brain MRI that indicated not only an MS lesion, which he failed to mention, but also a golf-ball sized meningioma, a benign brain tumor, on the right side of my brain. It took a while before the shock of this diagnosis would wear off and I'd wonder why a tumor on my right side would cause both feet to be numb.

"You *do* have MS," said the surgeon from whom I sought a second opinion on the tumor. I was scheduled for surgery the next day, and I was desperately looking for a sign that everything would work out. Days earlier, my rabbi warned me that having faith is a lot easier during good times than during bad. When I told him I needed a sign, he asked me what sort of sign I'd accept. I told him I couldn't think of one. "If your neurologist had run an MRI of your spine," the surgeon continued, "he would have found a lesion there. That's why your feet are numb. You have to have the tumor removed, of course, but once that's over, get an MRI of your spine and you'll see the lesion." Had Satan found the tumor because he arrogantly ran the wrong MRI? In that case, a series of events conspired to reveal a tumor that, while treatable now, would have led to seizures or even death had it been allowed to keep growing. Were this doctor's words the sign I sought?

"You don't have MS," said the confident surgeon who removed the tumor. "It must have been the tumor that caused your MS symptoms all along."

"Do tumors come and go?" I asked. "Because I had an MRI to diagnose the MS, and I've had MRIs since, but none of them showed a tumor until this one."

"No, tumors don't come and go."

"So I could have MS."

"I guess you could. You should see a specialist."

"You do have MS," said the kind neurologist. He seemed to be exactly the type of doctor I needed. He worked at the MS center one day a week, so he knew MS, but he worked as a general neurologist the rest of the week, so he wouldn't view everything through the lens of MS. He had given me a routine exam—I walked heel-to-toe, and he held a tuning fork to my legs—and asked what he could do for me.

"You can tell me why a tumor on the right side of my brain would make both my feet numb."

"Is that it?"

"Yes."

"I'll be right back." He had been examining my medical records and left to view my MRI. "You have MS," he said on his return. "Your other doctor must have been blinded by the meningioma. Look—you can see the lesion right here."

Another feet-numbing relapse six months later confirmed what my new doctor said—I do indeed have MS, and it's a good thing, for without it, I wouldn't have known about the tumor until perhaps it was too late.

> "When I think back on my latest neurological adventures, I am grateful that I have MS. If not, I'd be much worse off."

One of my favorite stories from Jewish tradition concerns Rabbi Akiva. Rabbi Akiva was traveling via donkey, with a rooster to wake him in the morning and a candle to help him see at night. He stopped in a city where no one would give him lodging. Rabbi Akiva continued on his way, responding, "Whatever the Holy One does, He does for the best." He continued to the woods and set up camp. That night, a lion killed the donkey, a fox killed the rooster, and a wind extinguished the candle. Rabbi Akiva, ever the optimist, reacted by saying simply, "Whatever the Holy One does,

He does for the best." The next morning, Rabbi Akiva learned that an invading army had captured the city. Had he stayed in the city, he would have come to certain harm. Had the army heard the donkey or rooster or seen the candle's flame, he would have been captured as well. As it turns out, Rabbi Akiva was correct: "Whatever the Holy One does, He does for the best."

I am not as much an optimist as Rabbi Akiva. Sometimes I don't think that things happen for the best. When I think back on my latest neurological adventures, however, I am grateful that I have MS. If not, I'd be much worse off. Do I ever lose sight of this lesson? Sometimes. Do I get frustrated with my MS? Of course. Then I feel the numbness in my feet, think of Rabbi Akiva, and smile. Sometimes things, even MS, do work out for the best.

Staci Bernard-Roth holds a Ph.D in English from the State University of New York at Stony Brook. A native Brooklynite and former Long Islander, she now resides near Atlanta with her husband and daughter. She teaches language arts at Parkview High School in Lilburn, Georgia.

A Short in the Cord

Joan Wheeler

When I was in the Air Force, I was fortunate enough to live "on the economy," which meant that I did not live in the base dorm, but had my own little apartment a few miles away. The furniture was eclectic and about twenty years old. There was one swing-arm lamp, harvest gold, which was attached to a piece of marble over the radiator. Nothing remarkable about this lamp: it would turn on and off, it would light the darkness, it matched the fuzzy gold cover on the chair in the corner. But one day, the lamp suddenly flickered off. Then it came back on. Sometimes it would just dim or flicker before popping on at the right brightness. Other times it worked fine. It was unpredictable and very irritating. I changed the bulb, I tapped the switch, I swung the arm all around, I banged on the lamp, I replaced the socket. Nothing worked. I later discovered that there was a short in the electric cord where it met the plug. The protective insulation around the cord's wire had been worn away, thus interrupting the electrical flow, shorting out the cord intermittently.

This story could also describe multiple sclerosis. Like the frayed lamp cord, with MS some nerves in my system have shorted out. And the symptoms of MS are as unpredictable as that living room lamp.

It was 1986; Reagan and Bush (Senior) were in the White House and the Communists were still the bad guys. I was married and living with my husband in a small duplex in Maryland. Out of the Air Force for five years, I was working for RCA and my desk was in the basement of a Defense Department building. One day, I felt a little light headed. I didn't think much about it, but it lasted for a few days. I took a break one morning and ventured to the first floor medical center and waited my turn to see a doctor.

Two doctors walked into my room and as they talked to each other, I suddenly flashed back to an old radio show called the *Bob and Ray-dio* Show featuring two guys who were pretty clueless and silly and very funny. Listening to these two doctors banter for a few minutes, I was convinced that Bob and Ray were seeing me. One looked up my nose and said, "Oh that's your problem." Then they started bantering again. They gave me antihistamines and sent me off scratching my head, wondering about the quality of medical care being given to the nation's Defense Department employees who were keeping us safe from those pesky Communists.

The antihistamines did not make me feel better, and the lightheadedness turned into dizziness. I later went to another doctor who referred me to a neurologist. By this time, I was in really bad shape and unable to work. I have vague memories of a CAT scan, of being injected with some contrasting material that made me shake uncontrollably. Inconclusive findings from the CAT scan led to an EEG. The results of the EEG were abnormal, showing that my central nervous system had gone berserk. The doctor thought that a virus that was attacking my nervous system. The end result was a prescription for a Dramamine patch that I put behind one ear to help the dizziness. This lasted for months.

Although my memories from that time are jumbled, missing, or confused, I remember lying on the couch watching T.V. Because of the recent Chernobyl nuclear reactor accident and the Cold War, the nation was paranoid about war and disasters. There were lots of horrific nuclear holocaust movies, shows and documentaries. Spending too much time alone watching those shows all day and not being able to stand up or go to work caused me to become severely depressed. I remember my husband's reaction: "Well then, just buy a gun and kill yourself now." He had no idea how close I was to doing just that.

It was 1993 and Clinton and Gore were in the White House. The Berlin Wall had fallen in 1989 and the Soviet Union had broken up (as had my marriage). I was dating again and working for a company called CSC as a quality assurance manager. In the previous year, Annette Funicello went public about her MS after rumors surfaced that she was an alcoholic, but I didn't notice.

While reading a book on a drive to visit my parents with my boyfriend, I noticed a tiny fuzzy spot in my right eye, and kept cleaning my glasses to clear it. A few days later, that fuzzy spot was still there and seemed to be getting a little larger. I silently panicked. I was terrified. Was I going blind? I was diagnosed with optic neuritis and started taking steroids. Nothing really serious after all, and I felt silly about panicking. I missed a few days of work and wore an eye patch for a few weeks, but eventually got back to normal.

In 1995, relations between the US and the former Soviet Union had warmed enough that the US space shuttle docked with the Russian space station Mir. But the federal building in Oklahoma City was bombed and Prime Minister Yitzhak Rabin was assassinated, confirming that there was still a lot of disruption in the world.

Disruption was about to erupt in my personal life as well. In March I had a fuzzy patch in my vision again, but I didn't panic this time. I knew what to expect and wasn't worried. I went to the eye doctor on my 36th birthday. I was nauseated from the jerkiness of my vision and was disappointed because I would not be able to go out to dinner for my birthday. After the examination, while the ophthalmologist was scribbling notes in my chart, he mumbled, "I'm referring you to a neurologist."

"Why?" I asked.

"Because you have MS," he blandly stated.

"What?" I cried.

"I thought you knew," he replied, and kept writing.

Happy birthday to me.

The next day I got a call from a kind nurse asking when she could come over to my house and hook me up for five days of intravenous steroids.

"What?" I cried.

"I thought you knew," she responded.

Apparently, some doctor ordered a five-day dose of steroids without telling me. I didn't comply because I was still reeling from the diagnosis and was in denial.

My visit to a new neurologist revealed that maybe I had MS, but maybe not. He ordered an MRI, but because I have a metal pin in my left ear (due to previous surgery) I was unable to have one. The neurologist said that he could do a spinal tap to confirm a diagnosis, but I might not have any more symptoms and this might be as bad as it gets. He explained that treatment for MS is an injection every day for the rest of my life, so unless I was willing to give myself a daily shot, I shouldn't get a spinal tap or have any other tests. Of course, I was not willing to give myself a shot everyday just to keep from wearing an eye patch every two years! That is how I became a "Maybe Baby"—maybe I have MS, maybe not—and stayed one for years.

In 1997, Princess Diana died in a car crash in Paris. Hong Kong was returned to Chinese rule. Dolly the sheep was cloned and Ellen came out of the closet. Clay Walker, country music star, was diagnosed with MS but I didn't notice.

My boyfriend and I, now living together, moved to Delaware in the fall—he took a job with CSC on the JP Morgan account and I took a job on the DuPont account. The move to Delaware was very stressful for me. Although I moved within the company, it was as if I joined a new one. Benefits were different. Rules were different. Language and acronyms were different. I went from the Department of Defense intelligence world to the commercial DuPont chemicals and paints and fibers world. I had no mentors, no friends, no support group. I was an outsider.

With all this stress, it was no surprise when I had a little tingling start in my feet, like they were falling asleep. I was also struggling with fatigue, so obviously stress was getting to me. But I explained it away as a consequence of not exercising or stretching or eating right. In the past, I used massage therapy to relieve tingling in my hands and arms, so I sought out a massage therapist at a chiropractor's office in Delaware. I made an appointment for the next week, but in a matter of days the tingling worsened, spreading up my legs and working its way to my waist. I felt like I was being jabbed with needles.

I had had a few years to think about my "Maybe MS" diagnosis, so I suspected there might be an MS correlation. From past experience, I felt that seeing the neurologist was a waste of time, so I started seeing a chiropractor. The massage and chiropractic treatment relieved the discomfort, but it was still unpleasant and difficult to walk. Fortunately, I was able to work from home in my new job. This "pins and needles" episode lasted over two months.

A few months later, I stumbled upon an MS support group online and learned that with the development of new "open" MRIs, some people with metal in their bodies were now able to have MRIs. I was advised by an MRI technician to find out the actual composition of the pin in my ear. If it was pure stainless steel I could have an MRI. I tucked that in the back of my mind for future reference. Maybe I would need that information. Maybe not.

In 1999, David Lander ("Squiggy") and Montel Williams went public with their MS diagnoses. The previous year, Richard Pryor received the Mark Twain prize for humor but his MS made him too weak to perform or speak. It was suddenly hard to ignore MS, but there was still nothing to be concerned about. Or so I thought. But the biggest stories of 1999 were the Y2K computer bug scare and the many doomsday predictions for the end of the millennium.

Earlier in the year my personal doomsday began to unfold. As I was pulling into the driveway of my home, I saw that the purple clematis growing around the mailbox were in full bloom. "How beautiful!" I thought. Then I hit the mailbox. I damaged it and wrecked the side of my car. I was quite stunned.

A few days later, I walked to get my hair cut at a salon near my home. After my cut was finished, I went to the counter to pay my bill when I felt my right toes cramp up. Just a little cramp. I tried to stretch it out and wait for it to relax, but it got a lot worse and became incredibly painful. Soon my entire foot and right calf were cramping and I was clinging to the counter to keep from falling.

> "Patients no longer hear, 'There's nothing we can do.'"

As the cramp climbed up my leg and continued climbing, I croaked some words explaining that I had a cramp and needed to sit down. I tried to get to a chair but didn't make it. I found myself on the floor in terrible pain as my right arm and hand went into spasm and my entire right side was contracting into the fetal position. I heard one woman say, "I'm a nurse," and I felt a towel under my head. I saw people over me but I could barely talk. I was terrified because this cramping had engulfed my entire right side including my heart, lungs and stomach, and I felt like I was being crushed. The nurse said that all my muscles were in spasm and she tried to massage my thigh and hand. After a few minutes, the cramping relaxed. I sat in the salon's waiting room for about a half an hour, then walked home, staying aware of soft spots in the terrain in case I cramped up again. I blamed the cramping on the stress from wrecking my car and didn't think any more about it.

But sitting at my office desk a few days later I felt the cramping again. I knew what to expect, so didn't panic like I did the first time. I got someone's attention and asked him to hold my hand and help me to the floor until it passed. It did so in about two or three minutes, but my co-worker was so shaken up he told my supervisor. It was no longer a secret that something was wrong with me.

I had never heard of anything like this and did not believe this was a symptom of MS, so I checked in with my chiropractor. He suspected a number of problems such as a magnesium or potassium deficiency, but said I needed to see a neurologist. So I called one and took the earliest appointment I could get, which was six weeks later. While I waited, the spasms continued to hit at unpredictable moments.

The neurologist ordered an EEG. During the test, the technician made me hyperventilate and I went into a spasm. But I had warned her about what to do if it happened and she came over and held my hand and talked to me until it passed. The neurologist jokingly said that it was very considerate of me to have an attack while hooked to the EEG because he was able to see that I did not have epilepsy.

I finally got an MRI (yes, the pin in my ear is stainless steel so is not magnetic) and a spinal tap. After months of tests, second opinions and various consultations, I received a positive diagnosis of Relapsing-Remitting Multiple Sclerosis. I was no longer a "Maybe Baby." I started on Copaxone, a daily injection of a non-interferon drug to slow the progress of the disease, and learned as much as I could about MS. Suddenly, all the strange attacks of the last 13 years made sense.

It is now 2009, and a lot has changed in ten years since my last MS attack and positive diagnosis. The 9/11 terrorist attacks changed the global landscape and sent the US to war in the Middle East; Hurricanes Katrina and Rita devastated the Gulf Coast in 2005; and Barack Obama was sworn in as President in January 2009. The economic crisis has sent most of the industrialized world into recession. People have lost homes, jobs, and hope for a secure future.

My own future plans collapsed in 2007 when I was forced into early retirement due to intractable fatigue caused by MS. Gone were my career and education dreams. I have transitioned from Relapsing-Remitting MS to Secondary-Progressive MS, which is characterized by a continuing decline in function without the dramatic relapse-recovery periods. After the attacks stopped, I experienced increasing fatigue and right leg weakness. I now walk with a cane and a leg brace when leg problems are bad, and I need daily naps. I even swallowed my pride and got a handicapped parking placard.

Since my first MS symptoms appeared, I've seen the decline of the Soviet Union, the disintegration of the Columbia space shuttle, the execution of Saddam Hussein, and the collapse of the stock market. But in the midst of these dramatic events, I've seen the explosive growth of MS research breakthroughs and significant improvements in diagnostic techniques. Gone are the days of doctors telling patients to quit work and avoid exercise. Patients no longer hear, "There's nothing we can do." There are now five injectable medications that are effective in slowing the progress of the disease, which is five more than were available when I had my first attack. Stem cell research and spinal cord injury research have provided clues to the MS mystery, and there are many MS drugs in the pipeline queuing up for future testing. This gives me great hope that a cure is coming in my lifetime.

Even though the economic and global cords may be shorting out along with my own, a strong current of hope in the MS community continues to flow unimpeded.

Joan Wheeler lives with her husband in Newark, Delaware. She is active in her Unitarian Universalist church and hosts an MS chat twice a month.

I Can Do Anything I Want ... Just Watch Me!

Gerard Chalmers

That New Year's Eve will always be cemented in my mind. Not because it was an extremely hot day, or the traffic moving from Newtown to Darlinghurst was unusually slow, or that the lorikeets that visited my balcony in the afternoons suddenly appeared there first thing in the morning. That was the day my life would change forever.

Two years before I was living in a small one-bedroom unit in Lewisham. The flat was a bit of a dump, really, but it was cheap rent and close to work. My usual Sunday routine was to get up, make coffee, sit on the lounge, light up a cigarette and ring my mother. Mum and I talked about normal things that a son who is close to his mother would talk about. This morning, though, I remarked to her that as we spoke I was rubbing my shin, but couldn't feel it. She replied, "I don't like the sound of that. If it continues, make sure you see someone." "Yes, yes, yes, mother," I said sarcastically, as if she was treating me like a child. We talked some more and then said goodbye. The day continued and I forgot about my leg.

A few weeks later came the annual dance party night and I was excited to be going. My partner wasn't going, and I looked forward to spending time with my friends. I met them at the gate of the showground, all charged up for a big night of dancing. We were sure to make memories that night! We moved our way through the pavilion and found our spot. The place was pumping and thousands of people had already filled the dance floor.

"Let's dance, people!" one of my friends shouted, and we moved our way towards the middle of the dance floor, threading through the enormous crowd. We found the perfect spot right under the mirror ball, where we all danced in a circle, laughing and carrying on. But something just wasn't right to me. Something felt rather strange: I seemed to have lost my rhythm! *I used to be a dancer*, I thought. *Just because you stop for a while doesn't mean you lose your rhythm, does it?* After trying and trying, I decided to sit the night out. I couldn't keep up. My friends insisted, "Hey, there's no party without you." But I knew that something was wrong. I ended up leaving the party very early, quite depressed and bewildered.

The next day I booked an appointment at the local medical centre. I described my symptoms to the doctor: that I couldn't dance, that there was numbness and a "pins and needles" feeling in my hands and legs and that I had become excessively tired. The doctor assured me that there was probably nothing to worry about and prescribed anti-inflammatory medication that, he said, would take the symptoms away. I went home a bit dazed, feeling as if it was all in my head. So I took the medication, and the symptoms disappeared.

A few weeks later I found myself on an apartment hunt. I looked for weeks and eventually found a one bedroom, right in the heart of Newtown. It was the tallest building in the city and, being on the fifth floor, had views of all of the city and right out to Parramatta. Bathed in sunlight and with a cooling breeze that went right through the unit, it seemed like home as soon as I walked in.

Things seemed to be going well for me. I was working long hours for an advertising agency, but enjoying the party life of a normal single person in his late twenties. But one evening when a colleague dropped me off near home, I had a frightening incident. Suddenly I couldn't coordinate my legs, and the walk became a nightmare. I arrived home in a panic. What was this, and why was it happening?

As much as I wanted to pretend nothing was amiss, I knew that something was wrong. In the coming weeks I had more trouble with my co-ordination, the pins and needles in my hands and feet came back stronger, and I even got asked to leave a pub because the bouncer thought I was intoxicated—when all I had was two beers! I would walk home from the train station after work, which was five minutes from my flat, and need to sit down for half an hour before I could do anything.

> "You have two choices in life. You can crumble or you can make the most of the opportunities that present themselves to you."

A friend recommended a well-known and thorough doctor. I booked an appointment and wrote down every effect I was experiencing: I wanted to get to the bottom of this. I kept thinking, am I going crazy? Am I making this up? I went to see her and told her of all the symptoms that I was experiencing. She booked me straight in to see one of Sydney's top neurologists. It was then that I knew something *was* happening to me. But the appointment was three long weeks away.

The next Thursday, I awoke with a strange feeling. As Thursday was our busiest day in the agency, I knew I could not ring in sick. I got dressed and went to work, still feeling strange. Things at work were, as usual, high-paced and stressful. At about midmorning I got up from my desk to take a job to the creative department and found my legs were not moving as fast as my upper body. I collapsed. I was sent to my doctor, who contacted the neurologist and shortened my appointment. I was told not to work until I saw him.

New Year's Eve was the day of my appointment. My mum and dad had come down from the Central Coast to Sydney for support. I had mixed feelings of nervousness and excitement. Maybe there was nothing wrong, or maybe there was just an infection that could be dealt with by antibiotics. The neurologist sent me for an MRI of the brain and spine. After the MRI, the neurologist asked us to join him in his office. He closed the door. "Gerard," he said, "the scans indicate that you have multiple sclerosis." The room went silent. I didn't know if I felt relief or confusion. But I finally had a "label" to pin on all the symptoms I had been experiencing and a reason to think that I wasn't as crazy as I thought.

It was decided to book me into hospital straight away for a lumbar puncture to take fluid from the spine area. If the fluid contained a high level of protein, then the diagnosis of MS would be confirmed. After the lumbar puncture was done, I would begin a five-day course of a steroid called methylprednisolone, which tends to prevent a relapse of the disease and boosts you pretty much back to normal. No one could tell me when and what exactly was going to happen next. I didn't even know what questions I wanted to ask. I felt like I was living in dream and that maybe the dream would soon be over.

I arrived back at my flat and rang my closest friend, Fiona, and told her of the news. "Do you know what MS is?" I asked her. There was a long pause, and then she replied, "Wheelchair... Isn't that what Betty Cuthbert has?" I said that it was, but only a small number of people with MS end up in a wheelchair, that part I knew. We spoke briefly and I left it to her to inform our other friends. I then had to rush to be ready for my hospital trip.

Over the next few months, it was hard for me to believe that I had a disease. Some days I wouldn't experience any symptoms at all. I decided that I needed to change my life; I needed a chance to put things into perspective. I left Sydney, to "downplay" my life and listen and pay attention to what my body needed.

Since my diagnosis, MS has become a major part of my life. I have spent weeks over these years in hospitals and in rehabilitation, learning how to walk again. I now use crutches. For years I refused to even look at a wheelchair; to me, it screamed "disability." When I finally got one, I could not believe the difference it made to my life. My love of shopping returned! I could go the distance of the shopping centre without feeling exhausted!

You have two choices in life. You can crumble or you can make the most of the opportunities that present themselves to you. I am not going to say that this has been easy. Every day I am met with challenges, both physical and emotional. But that's exactly what they are: challenges. Challenges that are there to be overcome. You will never hear me complain and you will never know if I am having a bad day. I remain as positive as I can and by doing so, try to portray this situation as a new beginning, not an ending. With the research that is taking place around the world, I believe that in my lifetime, we will see a cure and I will walk again.

Since my diagnosis, I have matured a lot and priorities have changed dramatically. One thing that has stuck with me is the importance and support of family. Without them, I could not have achieved half the things that I have. I live by one rule, one I hold deep in my heart:

I can do anything I want—watch me!

Gerard Chalmers resides on the central coast of Australia and is completing a Bachelor of Teaching degree and a Bachelor of Arts degree at the University of Newcastle to fulfill his desire to teach drama. He became an MS Ambassador to help raise the awareness of MS and the impact the disease has on the lives of people living with the challenge of MS. He always remains positive and looks for things to do in which he can challenge himself and surprise everyone else.

Part II
Now What?

Walking on Stilts

Cindy Lens

Entering the cavernous church a few moments before mass began, I made my way to the very last pew. Other spots closer to the front were open, but I chose to sit here, hoping to slip in unnoticed. Before I sidled into the old, hard wooden pew I raised the lowered kneeler, resting my forearm crutches between myself and a fidgety eight-year old towhead. Constantly popping from his seat, he strained to see the altar. As his mom pulled him back down, his gaze rose to the ceiling counting the chandeliers, only to pop up again seconds later. With each reposition, he picked up his chandelier count from where he last left off.

Watching the procession to the altar, the boy trembled in anticipation. I began to gaze in his direction. Happiness and curiosity were contagious. Grudgingly, I sat through many hours of Mass but this boy, bubbling with excitement at the coming event, made even me strain my neck a bit to see what was happening. Finally, his mom reached out, gently clasping his shoulder, pulling him back to the wooden pew for good. She motioned the universal sign for quiet, one index finger to the lips without even a "Shhh." Her arm draped around his shoulder, not as anchor but as loving embrace. Tossing him smiles, her eyes lit up whenever she glanced in his direction.

Surveying his immediate surroundings, the boy glimpsed my crutches. His eyes busily moved up and down the shiny metal sticks, then widening a little as he looked me over. I was still trying to get used to the stares of children; most held their eyes firmly on me as the rest of their bodies backed slightly away following their mothers' lead. From the corner of my eye, I saw his mom gingerly turn the boy's head to the center; all the while I could see the gears inside his head turning.

"Oh God," I thought, "This is the first time this little boy has seen a disabled person up close." I knew what was coming next: pointing, staring, questioning. Great! I had only recently starting using the crutches. Simply walking was becoming a burden. For 38 years, no one stared at me, but at age 39 I was diagnosed with multiple sclerosis. Struggling to adapt to my new condition, struggling to ensure my life was only changing, not ending, struggling to maintain a level of normalcy, independence became my life's work. The biggest change was the public perception of me. Being stared at for my good looks is one thing, but that never occurred. Being stared at because you walk funny, because you use forearm crutches is uncomfortable at best. I see most children just imitate the behavior of their parents. This newfound attention was more debilitating than the disease itself, robbing me of dignity and anonymity. The stares were invasions of my privacy, and that was the most difficult hurdle to overcome.

Tugging on his mother's blouse, he whispered into her ear. She blushed then giggled, squeezing his shoulders into her body. Now I stared directly at these two embracing, as her eyes met mine.

Looking at her son, she bent towards me while tousling his hair. "He's an eight-year old with a curiosity streak more than a mile wide." I nodded pleasantly in return, unsure where this was going. She turned around, motioning for the women standing directly behind us to join our tête-à-tête. Quietly trying to suppress the urge to stand, to yell about the improper response to someone who is different from you, or about the proper way to teach a child tolerance and acceptance, I inched towards the women, noticing the boy's now ruddy complexion. Struggling against the impulse to scream, "I am not different from you!" I hesitantly waited for this mother to speak.

"My son asked if after Mass you could demonstrate those stilts for him," motioning toward my crutches. "He thought the cuffs fit around your ankles while your feet rested on the handles," pausing for the imminent chuckle. "Quite a unique way of looking at things, don't you think?"

> "Surveying his immediate surroundings, the boy glimpsed my crutches."

Moving her eyes from me to the other woman as her free hand cupped her son's head, she said, "I thought you would like to know how your grandson's mind works." Smiles spread from mother to grandmother as we all moved back to our original positions.

The full weight of this boy's idea took time to settle upon me. Thrust into a new light through the eyes of an eight year-old, I was no longer in a defensive position. Moving freely from that day forward, I hold my head high as I demonstrate for all to witness how to keep your balance while walking on stilts.

Cindy Lens is the youngest of six siblings, half of whom have multiple sclerosis. She graduated summa cum laude from the University of New Hampshire with a Bachelor of Arts degree in English, and is now pursuing a writing career. Cindy resides in Amherst, New Hampshire with her loving husband, wonderful son and rambunctious chocolate lab.

What The People Don't Know

Judi Chatowsky

The ends of my nerves are frayed like a shoelace without the plastic tip. My brother's nerves are frayed, smashed, squished, sliced by bone shard, mashed into his spinal chord at T-12. It's a mess in there, or at least it was until the docs went in, cleaned things up, stuck in a metal rod and sewed him back together; Frankensteinian scars purple on his back. I still stare.

I was twenty-eight when a twelve hundred pound horse crushed my younger brother's spine. The night I found out, I lay on the cold tile floor of my basement apartment praying, bargaining with God like a child desperate for that special Christmas toy. But instead of vowing to be good, I was promising my legs—my own Isaac on the stone.

"God, Matt can't be paralyzed; he's an athlete, an outdoorsman, an adventurer. I can survive a desk job. I am surviving a desk job." I disintegrated into a swirling darkness, an altered state, prayers for my brother barely audible. When I came to, I wiggled my toes, my feet, my knees, both my legs. I could walk. Matt could not.

Two years after Matt's accident that left him paralyzed from the waist down, I phoned home to Florida from the University of North Carolina's emergency room. When Matt answered, I rattled off as much information as I could.

"Matt, I'm in the hospital, there's something wrong with me, I thinks it's my brain. I can't feel the left side of my body, I just got out of an MRI, I'm alone, half naked in this hospital gown, I'm freezing. Nobody's telling me anything and I'm stuck here with an I.V. in my arm. They want to do a spinal tap." I wasn't crying; I was frustrated.

"Jude, calm down. We don't know what it is. You're just going to have to go through it. Don't let any med students work on you."

That's it? I thought. *I'm in the hospital with a numb body, ready to get a twenty-inch needle stuck through my spine and all I get is, "You're going to have to go through it?"*

"Is Mom home?" I asked. She wasn't, she was out shopping. The doctors and nurses arrived.

"Matt they're here for the spinal tap. I'll call you when I get more news."

I was annoyed with Matt's Mr. Tough Guy, no emotions act. What about a little sympathy? Then I remembered that my brother, half conscious and unable to move, had waited twelve hours on a mountaintop in the Sierra Nevadas to be airlifted to a hospital. A sobering thought. My situation wasn't too bad, not bad at all, really.

I turned to face my spinal tap team. When I heard the medical student asking the attending physician if she had the needle in the right spot, I demanded more anesthesia. My case was textbook. My diagnosis: multiple sclerosis. In addition to the multiple brain lesions, the MRI showed a lesion on my spinal column at T-12.

Over the years, Matt and I have developed a comraderie around our respective disabilities. He's the one person who can tell me to "take it." On a winter day following my diagnosis, I woke with a severe case of vertigo. The art on my wall turned like a Ferris wheel. Sitting up made me nauseous. Unable to reach local friends, I called home. Matt, still recuperating at my parent's house, picked up.

"Matt, I can't sit up for very long, I can't walk without hitting the walls, I can't reach any of my friends, and I'm hungry." I whimpered. A moment of silence. Was Matt dismayed that he couldn't offer help?

"Jude, you got a phone right? You're calling me, right? Order a pizza pie. I have to do it all the time when I'm laid up with bed sores and I can't even roll onto my back."

"Oh, yeah, I guess I could do that; order a pizza pie."

Don't get me wrong, it's not always "buck up" with Matt. We commiserate, too.

"It gets hard for me, watching my friends do things I can't do anymore," I tell him, "Simple things, like staying up past 9:00 or spending time with their kids and then making dinner. I pass out when Bruce gets home from work. I feel like an old lady."

"I know Jude, I know. I don't even like being places where people are doing things I can't do. Believe me, I know."

Or we'll talk in code, using our favorite homemade pithy saying— "The people"—which is short for "The people don't know," and used in situations where someone, or everyone, is oblivious to the needs of the handicapped.

Two summers ago, when we were visiting Reno for my sister Amy's wedding, Matt and I decide to take a roll/stroll around the neighborhood. It was awful. The cracked and bumpy sidewalks ended without down ramps, forcing Matt to roll off driveways into traffic.

"Those mother f...ing...." Matt started.

"The people, Matt" I reminded him, "The people."

"Yeah the stinking people. I'm going back to the house."

He turned his wheelchair around and gave a high wave. I didn't take offense at being abandoned. Matt obviously had had it with being reminded that his legs don't move; he needed to cool down. Whenever we use this term, and believe me, it gets used a lot, I am reminded of a billboard strategically placed in the proximity of strip joints and biker bars on Route 19 in Tarpon Springs, Florida. A gigantic close-up of Jesus from the waist up, hands blooming with nails, head bleeding and encircled by thorns. Underneath, the caption screams, "Forgive them Lord, they know not what they do."

The people don't know, and I don't know, either. I don't truly know what it's like to live every day in a wheelchair. Matt and I have things in common (we both hate stairs) but I can't begin to know the day-to-day struggles of living in a wheelchair, and Matt doesn't understand the nuances of multiple sclerosis, a condition that remains, often frustratingly, invisible.

> "Over the years, Matt and I have developed a comraderie around our respective disabilities. He's the one person who can tell me to 'take it.'"

Matt has tremendous energy. Except for the times when he's weakened by a urinary tract infection or bed sore, he's up at 5:30 A.M. brewing coffee, whistling a tune, and he doesn't stop until bedtime. Except when I'm in a full-blown relapse, where my arms, legs, balance and vision are affected, fatigue is my most constant and debilitating symptom. The psychological and emotional implications of chronic fatigue are fierce. Coming from a robust family of eleven, where physical activity is given highest accolades (my parents, now in their seventies, recently hiked parts of the Appalachian Trail), I still feel guilty, bad even, because I am limited in what I can do or offer.

"No Wimps" brags the bumper sticker displayed on my mom's Suzuki Samurai.

Am I just being wimpy? Or is MS to blame? It's my fault I'm tired—I'm not eating right, too much sugar. I need more exercise. I'm staying up late, I'm bored, unfocused, uninspired. After ten years of living with this disease, I still fall easily into self-blame. I exhaust myself trying to figure out what I'm doing to make myself so tired. Self-validation and acceptance are a daily struggle.

"The people" don't know. They don't know that I'm so tired. They can't tell when I'm off balance and nauseous from vertigo. They can't see that the right side of my face is numb, my right hand and both feet, too. They don't know how draining a trip to the grocery store can be.

And they definitely don't know about the black hole (an actual medical term) in my brain, a spot where my nerve endings have died, leaving empty space. It's the abyss that names, dates, appointments, car keys, grocery lists, shoes, socks, pants etc. float into; a vacant stare left in their wake. Too many black holes cause brain atrophy, resulting in all sorts of problems, dementia for example. There are times when I walk around feeling like a three-headed, twelve-eyed, purple monster with warts.

I can't believe the people don't know, but they don't. "I don't even know," my husband tells me, "and I live with you."

It's been twelve years since Matt's accident and ten years since my diagnosis. I don't ache for him to walk any more. He's paralyzed, yes, from the waist down, but his life is full. Fuller even, than many ambulatory folk I know. On his last visit to my house in North Carolina, he helped me put in posts for a bicycle shed. Each morning when I returned from dropping my son off at pre-school, he would be waiting for me at the shed site; posthole digger, level, shovels, tamper, concrete and eighteen-foot posts scattered about. *Couldn't we just sit in the shade and talk about the bicycle shed?*

I thought as I put on my work pants. No way. We dug, measured, tamped, mixed concrete, and when I faded out after not quite two hours, Matt continued. By the time he left those posts were up.

My favorite part of that project was our conversation.

"Matt, I read in the National Multiple Sclerosis Society magazine that people with MS are better adapted to aging than their non-MS counterparts. Isn't that great news? I'm really pleased about that."

"Well, you already know how to use a cane," Matt quipped, as he bent over his chair with the posthole digger.

"I know one thing about aging for me."

"What's that?" I asked.

"It ain't gonna be pretty."

I stopped for a minute, shovel in hand, thinking about the implications of Matt's comment. I've never researched aging complications for paraplegics. I flashed on the "sensitive" neurologist who asked me if I wanted my three-year-old son to be changing my diapers when he was thirteen.

"Matt," I said, "you might think you know, but it all *Depends*. It really just all *Depends*."

"Yep," he grunted while he continued to dig, "it all Depends."

Who knows? "The people" sure don't and maybe we don't either. Maybe we just don't know.

Judi Chatowsky lives in Carrboro, North Carolina with her husband Bruce and their four-year-old son, Jonah.

From Fear to Gratitude

Lori Meyers

As part of my job with a local magazine, I write an annual story about the National MS Society's Gala and Luncheon. I interview several incredible women who work feverishly raising money for the South Florida chapter of NMSS. In sharing their stories, they invite me into their homes and into their lives and confess their personal connection to multiple sclerosis. I listen intently and when I write the story, I always leave out one very important detail: that I am one who receives the benefits from the hard work that they do, because I have multiple sclerosis.

Just after my 40th birthday, I did not expect to suddenly lose 80% of the vision in my left eye. As a healthy woman with no history of MS in my family, I couldn't make sense of what my ophthalmologist was telling me: she said I had *optic neuritis* (an inflamed nerve in the eye), which is often a precursor to multiple sclerosis. Somehow, the whole experience seemed surreal. Somewhat catatonic, I went on with my routine, using one eye while driving my two children to school, working at my part-time consulting job and carrying on as though everything was "fine." Other than my parents and my husband, I didn't tell anyone. That is how I coped. My denial helped me and I held onto it.

After the diagnosis was confirmed through an MRI, I still felt it imperative to keep my secret. I surfed the internet for information about MS and it only made me feel worse.

Although I spent the next several weeks receiving intravenous treatment for my eye, on the outside, I appeared "fine." I spent the next several months becoming harder on the outside than I ever thought I could be. But inside, I was hurting terribly and using every ounce of my energy to pretend it wasn't true. To this day, I don't know why I chose denial as my weapon.

My husband, Robert, was my strength, and my parents shielded me from my pain in any way they could. Although I had experienced several of life's speed bumps before, this crisis reached deep into my soul. How would I be different now? Could I accept the new identity that I'd been given, but didn't want?

This progressive disease for which there is no cure (and no known cause) would take its own course and I would live with the fact that there is no blueprint for the future. MS affects everyone differently, from those who are confined to a wheelchair soon after their diagnosis, to those whose cognitive abilities decline rapidly, causing them to give up their careers, to those who rarely, if ever, feel fatigue, numbness or tingling. I would learn to live with the constant uncertainty while at the same time never lose hope that there would be a cure in my lifetime.

My medication (a daily injection) would prevent the worse MS scenario and deter rapid progression and discomfort for me. During this time, I was lucky to have several individuals to offer me a kind word, an objective ear, or a good wish. I would never forget what they did for me in every detail. Like the day I walked into the workout room in my community gym (I tried to continue my routine then, even working out). I hopped onto the stationary bike and a woman close to my age asked what was wrong. I began to cry. I told her the truth. She comforted me and told me about a friend of hers who had MS and was doing well. She listened, and what she said to me was helpful. I thanked her profusely and later invited her to my home for lunch.

A few weeks later I walked into the same workout room. That day the room was empty, but sitting on the bike that I often rode was a worn book entitled, *Where is God, When It Hurts? A Comforting Healing Guide for Coping with Hard Times* by Philip Yancy. I felt like the book was waiting just for me.

> "How would I be different now? Could I accept the new identity that I'd been given, but didn't want?"

I did ask a rabbi that very question (Where is God when it hurts?) during this time, and he replied with wisdom that still gives me peace. He told me that God is in your family and your friends. Life is full of events that are not handpicked for us, they just happen. Our family and friends are there to help us through these times, he explained. I'm still not sure, but maybe that is when I changed my habit of holding in my bad news.

Dealing with this disease and daily life has inspired me to become more spiritual, and I have grown more content with everything I have been given. Eventually, I regained 95% of my vision through the incredible treatment I received. In time, I allowed others to support me, to console me, to let me cry and usually to laugh a little bit too. Somehow, I learned that security would be there again, but only when I could find it deep within myself.

Lori Meyers is a wife and mother of two who was diagnosed with MS in 2001. She dedicates this story to her husband Robert, who for eighteen years has been her rock.

Positives for Every Negative

Sherri A. Stanczak

Some of my fondest memories are of when my boys were very small. My three sons were at a wonderful age, and I enjoyed watching them take their first steps, listen to their first words and just being there through all of the cute little things they did.

When I turned 25, I was diagnosed with multiple sclerosis. I was devastated. But even though it hit me very hard, I believe it hit my family even harder. My parents went into denial, my boys didn't understand and my husband couldn't deal with it at all. In fact, two years after my diagnosis, I went through a very painful divorce. I felt like I was fighting a losing battle and fighting it alone. There I was, a single mother with three boys, living in a mobile home, no work experience, a terrifying illness and no money in the bank. Not to mention my husband's haunting words: "No one would ever want you with three kids and M.S."

But even though I was "damaged goods," my beloved kids needed me. So I pushed myself. Hard. Somehow I was able to always find some kind of a job. I worked full time and managed to get my sons to their ballgames, Boys Scout meetings, band practice, choir, and even played room mother on my lunch hour. God must have given me this unbelievable energy to keep going like I did.

Of course, I still had my problems. I got sick whenever my stress or fatigue became too much. I had to miss days or even weeks of work at a time whenever I had loss of vision or mobility. I worried about losing my job. Sometimes I did. My boys started going through puberty and their grades started slipping due to the divorce.

But, as challenged as my energy was, it really helped me to put as much of it as possible into the boys. Whenever we could, we went skating, swimming and to the park. Whenever I did have a few moments to myself, I kept up with my writing, and some of it focused on my children. I wrote poems or little stories about the first time I held them at the hospital, their first day of school, some of their ballgames, junior high, puberty. I found that writing down things that hurt me or upset me seemed to be good therapy.

Not long after my divorce was final, I found a very special man. Actually, he found me. I didn't think that I was much of a catch, since I was just a poor country girl who lived in a mobile home, with three boys and no money. Oh yeah, I had MS, too. It took me a long time to realize that he really did want to be with me. Mike lived over an hour away. A long distance relationship was hard enough, but I also had three boys who did not want to accept their mom being with another man.

> "God must have given me this unbelievable energy, to keep going like I did."

We dated for seven years before we got married. We waited to make sure my boys were accepting of the idea and that it was the right thing for us as well. And it was so right. Imagine, he married me in spite of my illness. He knew that one day I may not be able to work or that I may become disabled. That didn't stop him from loving me.

A few years ago, my condition became worse, with my vision and my mobility both going downhill. I had to start giving myself interferon shots three times a week to keep my condition stable. It was hard for me to give myself shots, so Mike would give them to me. He never hesitated to help me in any way I needed.

I eventually had to quit work and go on disability, which was very hard for me emotionally. But all that time at home gave me the opportunity to pursue my writing. Within the past three years, I have been published in more than 20 magazines, several newsletters and online publications. I have even had two books published.

When I was diagnosed with MS 20 years ago, it seemed like it was the end of the world. But I have tried to find the good in each bad situation. My motto for years has been, "There are two positives for every negative." The shots are a good example. Twenty years ago, we didn't even have any medication like those that I inject now. I am fortunate to have my husband give them to me. There are two positives right there!

My boys are now grown and we are all very close, a success story in itself. I am happily married, I'm a writer, I live in a nice home and I even have a few bucks in the bank. Things aren't always easy and every day isn't picture perfect, but things could definitely be a lot worse. MS did not stop me from achieving my dreams. In fact, it actually made me look at things differently. The sunsets are more beautiful because there were times I couldn't see them. My walks in the park with Mike are very much appreciated because there are days when I can't even get out of bed. I make sure to enjoy my good days, because I have had some bad days.

It has been a tough battle, but I have not given in to it. I am determined to fight. Last week, I got a call from the M.S. Society. My youngest son nominated me for the "Woman of Courage" award. I am in the top five finalists. After I cried for a while, I dried my eyes and I thanked God for giving me so much. Actually my family should get this award. I could have never made it without them. They have helped me make all of my dreams come true. They are my dreams.

Sherri A. Stanczak resides in Missouri and is the mother of three boys. She has previously published a book, *From the Heart of a Mother*, and has had published a number of articles in publications that include *Missouri Life*, *Heartland Boating Magazine* and *River Hills Traveler*.

When a Word Changes Everything

Martha Elaine Belden

Disease. I haven't been sure what to think since they told me I had one. You always think that if anything ever happened like this, it would be one big life-changing moment, never forgotten. I guess it kind of happened that way, but not exactly. Sure, I knew before then that something was wrong—my speech had started to slur a few days before, but I could still communicate, I had an appointment for an MRI and a neurologist—things were okay. Then, an hour later, nothing came out. I tried to tell Miranda about the great deal I'd gotten on the fudge pops I'd just bought at Albertsons and ... nothing.

What do you do when you open your mouth and nothing comes out? I started crying. But Miranda, being the sensible, "let's not panic" type, suggested sleep. "Maybe you're just really tired. If it doesn't help, we'll worry about it in the morning." Easy for her to say. But she had a point. It was 11 o'clock at night, after all. I decided there was no alternative but to follow her advice and got in bed. Sleep, however, was not my best friend. That night, every insane, self-pitying fear and thought passed over me. I thought, *This is it. This is the night I'm going to die and finally meet the God I've been talking to all these years.* But then I thought, *No, I don't think I'll be lucky enough to just die. The hospital. That's what'll happen next.* Tomorrow I would call the doctor and she'd put me in the hospital. We could get the tests done faster that way anyway. Good ... now ... sleep ...

Hospitals make things real for other people. I had known I was sick for months ... felt the strange sensation that my brain was somehow detaching itself from my senses. Now that I was in the hospital, other people knew I wasn't just imagining things. Not that I don't wish now that I had been, but it's nice to know I wasn't some hypochondriac seeking attention or something. Many people came to see me, and I loved that, too.

I've been at home for a while now, and my family's been taking care of me. Unfortunately, I don't really know how to feel about that. These days I don't know how to feel about anything, actually. I guess it's nice to have people wanting to help and insisting I rest; but on the other hand, I wish I didn't have to, and I slightly resent that they're telling me to. It's funny how when everything's fine, all I want to do is find time to do nothing. Now nothing's all I have to do, and I hate it. I don't really have the energy to do anything more than nothing, but my brain wants to, and it sucks.

If I sit really still and silent and don't think about how I can't feel my body, I suddenly feel normal, and I want to get up and run a marathon or call everyone I know to show them I can talk again. But then I move again or yell at my cat to stop using the chair as a scratching post, and I'm yanked back to reality. But I can be honest with myself, too. I know the truth. I never really wanted to run a marathon anyway. And if I really want to talk to my friends, I still can. So I go back to reading *The Great Gatsby* for my history class and secretly wonder if I'm wasting my time. There is still the possibility that people won't let me finish out the semester, and also that other possibility that I couldn't even if they do.

Now I'm back at school, and things are different. I guess I knew that everyone else's lives would go on as usual, but coming back and actually seeing it has been harder than I thought it would be.

I find myself getting so angry so often over the littlest things. Then I feel guilty, which leads me to feel even angrier because I think, *I shouldn't feel guilty! I'm the one who got sick!* The hardest part has been trying to believe that, through all of this, God is going to bless me somehow while I try to be happy for my best friend who just got engaged.

It doesn't make it any easier that at the exact time in my life when I need a best friend more than anything, Kat has become a mere acquaintance I hardly see or talk to. And when I do, we talk of nothing but her and her big day. I hate myself for my bitterness and envy. I mean, I'm the one who told her I'd keep my newfound depression and disease-ridden thoughts to myself because I didn't want to spoil her engagement (I even had to fight her on it). But no matter how hard I try or how angry I get at myself, I can't push the bitterness aside. All I can think is, *I just want one day ... one day with her when the topics of flowers and dresses and churches and cakes and ministers are forgotten.* And although I know this will never happen, at least not till long

> "I never really wanted to run a marathon anyway."

after her wedding is over and maybe not even then, I also realize that if I did get this "one day," then I'd want more because I know that, deep down, the thing I really want is for things to go back to the way they used to be, and that can never happen.

It makes me sad to go back and read all this and face how utterly self-centered and pitiful I was (probably still am). I'm not dying ... my hair isn't even falling out ... and most of the time I can still do everything I used to. I wish more than anything that acknowledging there are so many people in the world so much worse off than I am, acknowledging how blessed I really am, would make all the pain and anger go away. But it doesn't. It just makes it worse, because then it's all magnified by guilt for feeling sorry for myself when really I should just buck up and move on with my life like everyone else has.

I know this will happen eventually. I know that one day I'll wake up and not even think about the fact that I have MS, and I'll later realize this and finally know that I have moved on. I know one day I'll probably have the attitude that shouts, "I will live my life! I will not let MS get in my way!" The problem I have with this is, I just don't know when that day will come. And right now, all I really want to do is hit those people. They make it sound so cheesy—like a commercial for genital warts or something. And besides, I'm not "letting" MS get in my way. It does that all on its own. Believe me, if I could wake up with tons of energy and feel motivated to live life the way I always have, I would do it in a heartbeat.

But I'm sure, one day, I'll move on and pick up that positive attitude that so many others seem to have.

Martha Elaine Belden is a 28-year-old writer living in Dallas, Texas. Diagnosed with multiple sclerosis during her senior year in college, she earned a Bachelor of Arts degree in English from Texas Christian University in 2003 and has been writing for national and international periodicals ever since.

Disability Blues

Dennis Fox

Emily's screeching on her recorder this morning fouled my mood even before I got out of bed. Shouting her name three times to quiet her didn't help. Too wired to sleep, too irritated at my irritation to face the day, I sank back, trying to remember if I had really been more patient two decades ago, when I'd first had six-year-olds, or if that memory, too, is distorted.

The doctors tell me the irritability is probably a multiple sclerosis symptom. The same for the immobilizing fatigue, mild depression and short-term memory loss. My sporadic loss of verbal fluency is also common to MS. But I'm not so sure. These problems come to everyone, my aging friends reassure me. "I forget things all the time," they say, impatiently. Things fall apart at 50, disabled or not. I don't haul out my MRI to insist, "Yes, but...."

My wife, working neither of her two jobs today, just asked if I want to go to a movie. With our daughter at school, we could avoid a babysitting fee. "I don't know," I mumble unhelpfully. To return from a movie early enough for my nap, I'd have to cut short my writing time. I feel pressured to produce more—Elizabeth can't work two jobs forever—and I'm distracted too easily.

As MS goes, I have it easy. Except for increased exhaustion, I haven't deteriorated since my diagnosis, seven years ago. The visual distortions, perhaps originating in the same sputtering part of my brain that caused my initial double vision, don't last long. There's no motor impairment yet—no wheelchair, no cane, no leg numbness or cramping except sometimes in summer heat. Some yoga poses leave me wobbly, but other students wobble too. I can walk on level ground for a couple of miles, just a little slower than I used to.

Often I feel healthy, just confined, pressed for time during my few good hours. To outmaneuver the fatigue, I've cut down on most things that wear me out. I don't walk as far as I'd like. I avoid the sun when it's past 75 degrees. I can still choose to push myself, to walk and do yoga in the same day, to stay up too late. The cost is being more drained than usual that day and the next. But I have the choice. I just wish I could dance for more than a minute or two when Emily turns on the music.

> "We may never climb mountains together as I did with her now-grown brothers, but I'm teaching her chess."

At the university, I heeded my doctor's suggestion: "Take it easy. Avoid stress. If it was me, I'd quit every committee I was on." Tenured, I could afford to stop working late every night, and ignore my dropping publication rate. I went to fewer conferences and campus meetings, rejected invitations to collaborate on new projects. When even a reduced teaching load became too difficult, I let that go too, and applied for disability leave.

The irony? As an academic, I had studied disability evaluation. How does the government distinguish someone who can't work from someone who doesn't want to? I had worked for the Social Security Administration in the seventies, interviewing applicants for benefits, and later for a state agency, deciding if applicants were legally disabled. So I knew that disability decisions are less certain and more subjective, more political, than any agency would admit. And I knew that asking the state's university retirement system to declare me "unable to perform my regular job" when I didn't look disabled, and didn't always feel disabled, raised certain complexities. At least I didn't have to meet Social Security's stricter standard: unable to perform any job at all.

My case dragged on—a cane would have helped, just for show—but they finally approved my claim. Otherwise I'd still be trying to fake my way through the workday, becoming the stagnant professor I never wanted to be.

I sometimes get jealous when friends take on new tasks, move to more interesting jobs, make the most of their prime earning years, while I putter around, calling myself a writer, estimating how poor I'll be when my benefits run out. Back in my twenties, when people like me didn't put aside money for the future, I supposed I'd work as long as I had to. I didn't have a fallback plan. Today, there aren't many job ads for "part-time work, mornings, not much energy required, decent pay."

I'm glad my condition's invisible, with my two-hour nap private, my easy limpless walk public. But when an acquaintance wonders why the sabbatical he presumes I'm on is now in its third year, I lack an honest response that doesn't discomfit both of us.

I think back on my days evaluating disability cases. It was easier writing about disability when I wasn't disabled. Three hours after sitting down at the computer my workday's mostly over, my grumpiness dissolved. I think I'll go for a walk, and then nap before Emily gets home. We may never climb mountains together as I did with her now-grown brothers, but I'm teaching her chess. As long as she stops screeching that recorder, I can still concentrate enough to hold my own.

Dennis Fox is now retired from his position as Associate Professor of Legal Studies and Psychology at the University of Illinois at Springfield and lives near Boston. He writes personal, political, and academic essays which have been published in *Salon*, the *Boston Globe*, *Education Week*, *Tikkun*, *American Psychologist*, *Law and Human Behavior* and other outlets.

Part III
Living with MS

A Country Named MS

Diane J. Standiford

One day I moved to another country. Not knowing the spoken language, not familiar with the foods of choice, and knowing no one else who had ever been to this place, well, I was on my own. The country was called Multiple Sclerosis.

Knowing I was headed either there or to the island of Brain Tumor, I was quite happy to have an MRI reveal my new path. Winding through symptoms including numbness, foot drop, legal blindness, slurred speech, fingers to feet that stopped functioning, I settled into my current life with twists and turns more dramatic than any rollercoaster. I was a long way from Indiana.

First I had to learn the language. MRI, ABC and sometimes RTN, NIH, CNS, RR, PT, OT, AFO; oh dear, hard to learn a new language as an adult, especially when the natives often speak in acronyms. The cuisine took some getting used to as well: green tea, low fat, lots of fruits and vegetables, high fiber, water galore. Out were my trips to Burgerland, fried chicken and frozen TV dinners. Oh, and for dessert: stretching with yoga and a thick topping of meditation.

The political system is not that unusual. Doctors, Researchers, Therapists, Pharmacists, all adding their individual ideas for a better MS. We do not vote, but we visit them and choose which ones will represent our needs the best. Sometimes they exceed our expectations; sometimes they drift off point, leaving us adrift as well. Fundraising is ongoing and there is never is enough money to deliver what we all want: a cure.

> "Each day is a new adventure, a new word to learn, a new fellow citizen to meet, a new mountain to climb."

We need not feel alone though, for there are societies, associations, and many groups that offer power in numbers. Thank goodness the Internet thrives in this country and offers engines to take us to many helpful sites. And since any miniscule point on any tiny nerve from the top of our heads to the tips of our toes can be compromised at any moment, well, no two bodies ever experience exactly the same physical mishaps, nor for the same length of time. No wonder the first pilgrims to this country were considered insane.

I guess the most difficult obstacle I had to learn to deal with was the uncertainty of life here. Oh, sure, in Indiana we had 10 degrees below zero and snow that stayed for months. Spring would bring tornados and the summer brought humidity with 90 degree temps that were unbearable. "Just wait and the weather will change," they used to say; actually that was said in my second home, Seattle as well. The same is true with MS: it's unpredictable and dismantles a goal-oriented planner like me.

Do not bother looking for a visitor's bureau; none exists, probably due to having to update brochures so often. (The cause is this; no it's not. Don't eat dairy; dairy is fine. It is not inherited; yes it is. This drug is best; no this one is better.) Besides, who would want to visit here? Better to lose your money in Vegas than to lose your mind here. Our brains are shrinking, atrophy of limbs sneaks up on us. No beaches for sunbathing or saunas for visitors, the heat will slow our nerve signals to a virtual stop.

Numbness, tingling, pain and spasticity are always nearby in this country. Weakness, depression, constant worries about the "f" word lurk around every boarded up tourist attraction. F for future, the fear one dare not say aloud. Jobs are so difficult to keep here. Money is always a concern and no insurance will cover our "pre-existing condition."

So I decided to embrace my new country, "go with the flow," "chill out," "take it one day at a time." After all, this is my home now. Each day is a new adventure, a new word to learn, a new fellow citizen to meet, a new mountain to climb. Yes, MS is my new home. I embrace the new person I have become and I wouldn't live anywhere else. Headed this way? Be brave, it is a great adventure.

Diane J. Standiford is a 50-year-old cancer survivor who lives with MS and attempts to bloom where she is planted. She is an advocate for people with disabilities and enjoys writing and making people laugh. Her true stories have been published both locally and nationally.

A Hot Day In July
Rachel Oliker, M.D.

Who would have thought that at the mature age of 36 I would be accompanied by my parents to the neurologist's office, just like doctor visits when I was elementary school-age? I usually like to venture into New York City on my own, but this time was different. I needed them with me. I couldn't walk independently because I was undergoing a worsening of my multiple sclerosis symptoms, or an exacerbation. I packed my prayer book and cell phone while my mother prepared a green apple—my favorite—and some cherries. It's times like these that assure me royal treatment, which always includes my mother's Russian cooking. But it's also times like these when I wish I didn't need it.

It all started with a pain in my left buttock a few weeks before, after a series of heat waves, with temperatures climbing above the 100, and the timely breaking of our air conditioner. I was living with my parents after years of study and medical school. What does a med student think of a pain in the ass? I'll ignore it, I reasoned, or perhaps massage it, hold it with my left hand. Holding makes a difference; after all, all ailments like to be held. My aunt, observing me clutch the area, suggested, "Why don't you make an appointment with your primary care doctor?" I was a little irritated by her suggestion. After all, I had been a medical student and

I knew what I was up against. Eventually, though, I had to give in when the exacerbation grew worse.

My father dropped my mother and me off at the hospital entrance in New York City,and. I tried to lose my worries about the coming appointment by observing the many people who patiently waited with us for the elevator: residents with proudly-displayed name tags and anxiety-ridden faces, attending physicians with faces full of contemplation, a mother with three subdued young children, visitors with flowers and expectant, glowing smiles, and maintenance staff, holding cleaning supplies. We finally squeezed our way out and proceeded to the neurology outpatient clinic, which was surprisingly empty of patients.

My father, dressed casually from straw hat to sandals and white socks, entered at the same time as Dr. Vorobei, a young, slim and smart-looking neurologist with a bow tie. After introductions, the doctor sent us across the hall to Laurie. We quickly get down to business. Laurie sat at the computer across the room and consulted my medical history and the record of my former appointments.

"Are you still swimming?" she asked. "Doing yoga, pilates, tai chi?"

"Yes, yes, yes, but not tai chi anymore," I answered. "And pilates only when I have access to the women's gym," I thought about it for a moment, and marveled at how a person can coordinate all these activities into a daily schedule, even when dealing with the trying symptoms of MS. Oh, the fringe benefits of being on disability!

"How about supplements? Calcium, vitamin D?"

I paused with a sense of guilt. "No, I don't take those anymore. Oh, I take a multi that has them, but in a lower dose."

All this was transmitted to the doctor. When Dr. Vorobei walked in, he got a quick debriefing from Laurie. His brow furrowed when Laurie ratted on me with gusto regarding the calcium and vitamin D. "Why don't you take those anymore?" he demanded, glaring at me. Swallowing hard, I replied, "I, I ... um, well, I was hoping to obtain all those vitamins from food," not really believing my own words.

He gestured with his arms wide open, "But you've lost weight; you look like you're on a starvation diet! Besides, you'd have to eat pounds and pounds of broccoli to obtain even a fraction of the required amount of the vitamin. So you should buy supplements with 2000 mg of calcium and 1200 mg of vitamin D." He went on, scolding me, "You know even taking vitamin D alone is good for MS. It helps with balance. Remember, we discussed this last time?"

He then performed the neurological exam, with my parents watching with curiosity from the other end of the room. My legs were weak. My balance was impaired, as demonstrated by my faulty standing and brief failed attempts at hopping on either leg.

Dr. Vorobei then left the room, leaving my parents and me to await Laurie's delivery of a a steroid injection. My mother took this opportunity to

> "Oh, the fringe benefits of being on disability!"

address the issue of my weight and nutrition and started spinning menu options on the spot, claiming that I could easily stand to gain 20 pounds, 10 at the very least. It was a disgrace for a mother of Russian origin, she insisted, to have a daughter who was underweight, and less than 100 pounds at that. She mapped out a filling cooking extravaganza—borscht for cleansing and increasing my blood count (so she said), beet salad, gefilte fish, potato pancakes, leafy green vegetables for iron, chicken and a Russian salad of chick peas, potatoes and green peas. How fortunate am I. Who could complain at this imperial treatment?

The steroid arrived; Laurie inserted the catheter into the vein in my right antecubital region. It hurt on its way in, and I looked

away. Even with the M.D. by my name, I still cringe at the inser-
tion of needles and other devices into my body. Before the steroid
started to drip, Laurie measured my blood pressure: 100/65 mm
Hg. The I.V. drip went smoothly and Laurie sat with me for a
while, discussing why my parents weren't as excited about my
upcoming trip to California as I was. I told her that I am supposed
to meet up with a guy and some other friends who live there.
Laurie's eyes perked up. "Let me guess," she said. "'No one is
good enough for our daughter.'"

"No, not really," I responded, remembering my parents usual half
joking/half serious query about any male I may describe: "What
disability does he have?" It's not an unfair question. My MS is
never far from my mind or theirs, and I'm sure they think I would
be better understood by someone living with his own challenges.
But I didn't explain this to Laurie. Instead I continued, "He's a
psychiatrist."

Laurie's eyes lit again. "Another doctor. Wow." Then she left me
with the I.V. flowing into my vein for another forty minutes. My
parents returned, bringing avocado sushi, which I ate with great
relish using my unfettered hand. The steroid infusion ended, but
there was no sight of Laurie. So my parents and I waited impatiently, while I began to get nostalgic about my medical degree and
its lack of implementation. I remembered my love of working in a
hospital. I missed it and the times I spent working with patients.
My parents argued that I didn't miss it or shouldn't miss it. But I
did, and I do. I thought of the many people less fortunate than I
am. MS patients who would not be discharged, as I was about to
be, for a pleasant ride home with my parents to a sumptuous,
home cooked Russian meal. Patients whose terrible symptoms
would cause them to stay many days and nights in the hospital.

Later, we headed back to the garage where my father parked the
car. My mother offered to hold my hand, but I argued that it
looked too childish. It was bad enough feeling helpess without

looking it. She still offered her arm in any case, and I took it reluctantly for stability, since I was limping. *Thirty-six and leaning on my mother*, I thought. Then I felt a flash of gratitude to have my parents with me.

The car came, we headed onto FDR Drive, and left New York City behind.

Dr. Rachel Oliker was born in Riga, Latvia, and moved to Jerusalem, Israel at the age of two. She pursued undergraduate studies at Stanford University in California, followed by a fellowship program in Israel. She earned her medical degree at the State University of New York at Stony Brook School of Medicine.

Feeling Numb

Jessica Lipnack

"I think I need to go to the Emergency Room."

"I need to go to the Emergency Room."

"Take me to the Emergency Room."

It is Saturday and there is no neurologist. When he arrives the next day, I drench him with questions. In the great divide of doctors who talk with patients and those who speak to themselves, this man stands with the self-conversers.

"What is wrong with me?"

It's a question larger than he can answer. And so it goes for the next ten, next twenty years. Spells of numbness so thick that I cannot feel my feet, bouts of fatigue that disturb my sleep and confine me to bed, stretches of bone-splitting agony that no medication, over-the-counter or prescribed, relieves.

I see several more chiropractors, leaving them behind when one, an ugly man old enough to be my father, slobbers a kiss over me. I see homeopaths: the first uses the word "weird" when I describe my symptoms; the second prescribes tablets made from snake venom. His office smells like rotting food; a few months later, I read that he has died.

I try no-fat, low-fat, fruits-and-vegetables, soy-free, and soy-based diets, consume so many supplements I worry I will grow fat from those alone, test my allergies and learn that I have sixty-three. I yank the mercury fillings from my mouth, run Vitamin C through my veins to flush the toxins, fast for ten days. I relinquish close to ten thousand dollars, spending nearly a month of my life with needles stuck in my meridians.

All that and more in search of relief, in search of a name, a cause for my ills. In the end, I owe my diagnosis to an MRI I get because of a migraine that lasts twenty-three days in a row.

"Nothing to worry about," the doctor says, meaning no brain tumor because every time anyone has a brain MRI that is the unspoken subtext.

"Send me the results, please."

And there, in black-and-white, "Lesions consistent with MS."

"Don't worry about it," my forever neurologist says, forever because he always encourages me, tells me to travel even in the midst of attacks, compliments my reflexes, tells me how healthy I look when I do, helps me down the hall when it's hard to walk, shows up at my house with a florescent light affixed to a headband that he wants me to wear when I fly to Tokyo because jet-lag will be very bad for me, calls me his poster child for what is possible with MS.

He takes a sample of my spinal fluid and measures the velocity of my nerves, an old-fashioned test invented by a doctor at his hospital.

"You have MS," he says, as I join my voice to others who say, "It doesn't have me."

It was thirty-odd years ago that I woke to a sparkling June sun and a body completely numb from my rib cage to my toes. It started that suddenly, without a yellow light or a distant oncoming horn, and another two decades would pass before it had a name. For all of my adult life, this MS, this disease whose insidious symptoms have never been completely captured by even the deftest of writers, has been my companion, coming without warning, decking me, then leaving just as fast. MS. Multiple scarring. I look up the definition a hundred times, chant the words like a mantra in a foreign tongue.

My symptoms *du jour*: changes in sensation, depression, severe fatigue, overheating, and pain. Numbness and its odd twin, tingling, but not the pleasant kind. A fifth of my left hand heavy, as if in a press, for a dozen years now. Long spells of deadness in my torso, a short walk too long for my falling-asleep legs. Tingling also in my vagina, where normally desirable, but not like this. My abdomen, my calves wrapped tighter and tighter, as if an ace bandage were pulled to its limits, until I fear I will implode. My central nervous system, plugged into a socket, sizzling, fraying, about to short out at any moment, and then, in the next, drained of all physics, every hidden erg suctioned dry.

I draw the nervous system, pen the fine lines of a dendrite, trace my frayed left ulnar nerve, magnifying the crevices where the myelin has gone missing. I swim through my brain, circle the plaque, stare down the black holes of lesions and pray they remain this benign. I pour buckets of white light over my head, wrap blue silk along my spine, bathe in a bag of oxygen, tap my inner power plant when I cannot lift my head, and eat no fat. Or gluten, root vegetables, meat, dairy, soy, and nuts. It is crazy-making.

Thirty-odd years of this, coming and going, confining me to bed, dropping me into a chair when everyone else stands, the telephone too heavy to hold, the Wall of Pain so impenetrable no forward step is possible.

Then, suddenly, nearly a year ago, I am better. It's loosened its grip, perhaps forever. Don't say that, friends warn. Bad luck. You'll have to eat your words. They are right, of course. Sheets of numbness, strikes of pain, dripping and drooping when the temperature rises, and my left hand is still numb. But, in the center of my being, I am well. Nearly a year. Unpredictable, my myelin, in its disappearing, its ravaging, and its reparation.

Thirty-odd years and now it is my sixtieth birthday and I'm eating sushi with my closest friends, gulping down *toro* even though I know it's heavy with metals. I say I feel better than I have since I was twenty-seven. They ask why.

> "MS. It cometh and it goeth."

The truth:

I read a book about back pain with a familiar message—bodies somatize emotions—and I decide I can feel better even when I feel worse, that I have choice.

I complete the novel I've wanted to write for thirty years.

I go back *on* gluten, eating pasta, bread, and more pasta, start drinking wine.

I go to physical therapy for "writer's neck;" hire a trainer.

I walk a few miles five of every seven days, travel to Europe and New Zealand and Alabama and Vermont in just under nine months.

I move my study from the third floor, where I can only see one tree, to the first, where I look onto the garden.

And as I write these words, my shins are flush with tingling, my left hand is still heavy on the keys, and the mist of fatigue is not far away.

MS. It cometh and it goeth.

Jessica Lipnack is the co-author of many books and articles. She heads NetAge, a boutique consulting company that advises global companies, governments, and NGOs.

Telling the World
Terry L. Wahls, M.D.

When I learn that I have multiple sclerosis, I ask about my long term prognosis, but the answers are vague: It's an unpredictable disease. Some do well. Others experience a relentless downhill course. There is no cure. Injections might decrease the number of MS flareups and slow the rate of accumulated disability. They cost almost a thousand dollars a month and are only 30 percent effective. But having many favorable signs, I am told, I will probably do quite well.

Because I'm a physician, and wanting to know more, I log onto PubMed. What I learn is depressing. Within ten years, half of all MS patients require assistance walking. Furthermore, half will be disabled, unable to work. I need to believe I'll do better, and start treatment. Every morning I run, take my injections, and go to work building a new Ambulatory Care Department. Work goes well, and my family prospers, enjoying the new opportunities available in a university town.

Like many with chronic illness, I want to deny I that have MS. But eventually, running becomes difficult. I put in a pool and switch to swimming each morning. My strength slips further away. Evenings I am tired. Back pain increases and I have more trouble walking. Others begin to notice. Initially I shrug off the inquiries about my limp, referring to prior sports injuries. I am tired by 2 P.M.; swapping out my desk chair for a chemo chair decreases my fatigue.

My doctor gives me a prescription for a brace, which I keep discreetly hidden under long socks and trousers. A few months later, he gives me a prescription for a scooter. When he changes his mind, telling me it would be better to get a wheelchair, I am even more dismayed. Am I really going down that fast?

What will I say at work? John, one of my staff physicians and also a good friend, offers to help. "I could mention you have MS in the office. It would not take long for the news to get through the whole department." Yes, it would be easier, but I tell him that it wouldn't right. The next day I have a staff meeting which includes our remote clinics, listening by phone. "On Friday, those of you who are on the main campus will notice that I will be using an electric wheelchair to get around the facility. I need it to manage the fatigue related to multiple sclerosis." As I speak, I see the shock and concern on their faces. Apparently my attempts to hide the MS has worked, my staff really had not known. "It should not have a major impact on the department."

One by one, the physicians come to talk with me.

"I had no idea."

"You look so good."

And then the difficult questions come.

"Who will lead the department now when you can't?"

"How much longer do you think you will you be able to keep working?"

"I plan to continue to work and run the department," I respond. "Nothing should change. It'll be fine."

If I want to continue leading, I must project confidence about the future. My heart is not quite as confident as the words I use, but I repeat them often anyway.

On Friday the wheelchair arrives. Now everyone knows, not just my department. Continually, I must answer their questions.

"What happened to you?"

"Are you okay?"

The first few times, I take people to my office to explain. With practice, speaking becomes easier. By the end of the week, I answer questions about my MS in the hallway.

I find that driving with a joystick is not easy. Making clinic rounds, I stop to speak with the scheduling clerks, driving my wheelchair to join them behind the counter. As I back away, I catch their desk with my chair. Try as I might, I keep making matters worse. The clerks need to help get my wheelchair disentangled from their desk.

"I guess you'll need to watch out for me. As you can tell, my driving is not yet the best." I laugh and so do the clerks. Laughing together, they can see I am not defeated. The story spreads, as does my confidence.

> "Choosing laughter again and again, my confidence grows. My future again looks bright."

Those first few days, when I say over and over, I will be fine, I begin to believe. Choosing laughter again and again, my confidence grows. My future again looks bright. I receive so much healing from those interchanges; I think *why is it we are not teaching our young doctors about the healing power of laughter?*

Dr. Terry Wahls is the Associate Chief of Staff at the Veteran's Administration Iowa City Medical Center and an Associate Professor at the University of Iowa Carver College of Medicine. She teaches Internal Medicine residents, performs research and sees patients. Diagnosed with multiple sclerosis in 2000, she is now completing her memoirs, detailing the challenges of becoming a physician, a single parent, and then being diagnosed with progressive multiple sclerosis.

Get a Room
Anita Stienstra

Bed is a great place to connect with a spouse, but not only in a sexual way. I am referring to laughter, conversation, activity, and lying close together. Quality time in bed with my husband has actually sustained our relationship through the struggles we face with multiple sclerosis. Early on, when Mark first started using a wheelchair because of spasticity and weakness in his legs, and when my role as caregiver had just begun, we often found bed a refuge. The combination of laugher and close proximity to one another made many nights and mornings more intimate and memorable.

One such night we lay secure in each others' arms and again played a silly game we had concocted. We positioned our nostrils close and breathed in and out in opposite union so his exhale filled my inhale, and his inhale filled my exhale. This ridiculous ritual brought on from our interest in yoga and meditation made us feel joined and complete. After months of performing it, though, we roared with laughter when the notion came to mind that perhaps we were only breathing in each other's carbon dioxide and perhaps poisoning each other. Then, we chuckled even more deducing that our laughter was probably oxygen deprivation. This single incident became a great bond between me and my husband. It is proof that one doesn't have to travel to exotic lands to share bonding experiences.

After about five years of life with MS, Mark and I began two other activities in bed. Reading became difficult for Mark—his eyes would bounce around the page—so we watched movies and I read aloud to him. The secret to getting the most out of these activities is to discuss the film you see or the book you read, and furthermore, to use the content or discussion as a catalyst to explore the smallest or largest of topics in different ways. For example, when we viewed *The Madness of King George* we were inspired to go on an internet quest to learn the history of King George III's reign in Great Britain. We learned that his behavior was caused by mental illness brought on by what is generally thought today to have been a blood disease called porphyria, the symptoms of which can at times mimic or exacerbate an unbridled passion and joy for life. He was one joyful fellow even if everyone thought him mad or if he was indeed mad.

> "Laughter and being silly were and still are good medicine for us."

Mark and I soaked up King George's zest for life and love for his wife, Queen Charlotte. We mimicked a scene in the movie every night when going to bed, where the king and queen tell each other, "Goodnight Mr. King. Goodnight Mrs. King." We changed the phrase to, "Goodnight Mr. God. Goodnight Mrs. God," because we have a friend with the last name of King. This exchange of words became our bedtime ritual. It was childish affection but laughter-producing every time. Laughter and being silly were and still are good medicine for us.

Tennyson states in his poem *Memoriam*, "'Tis better to have loved and lost/Than never to have loved at all." Similarly, Mark and I believe that it is better to have loved and laughed and lost, than never to have loved and laughed at all. Particularly with MS. It is hard to have fun in the face of ever-changing and dire circumstances. Mark has been Heimliched four times. Sometimes it is hard enough to remember to have fun as adults, let alone as adults dealing with disease. No matter how challenging a wheelchair can be, or facing the daily deterioration of range of motion and decreased function from fatigue, these moments help us forget and feel good before other taxing situations arise.

If you need an exercise to help loosen you up, I suggest the tai chi laughter exercise. How it works in a tai chi group is that everyone forces himself to laugh for three minutes. The forced laughter at the beginning of the exercise produces real laughter after a while, and in turn everyone laughs even harder from hearing true and unique giggles and hoots. This is a great exercise for everyone and can be easily done in bed. I am not suggesting that all bad moods need to be immediately eradicated. At times sadness or anger need to be embraced and worked through. But if you've become disconnected with a loved one or negative feelings have persisted for too long, try snuggling in bed again. Try laughing in bed again. Try finding an activity in bed where you are relaxed and close to each other. Don't stop trying.

Recently, my stress level increased to the point that the laughter and bedtime activities began to decline. Most of the time we fell wearily asleep the moment our heads touched the pillow. I had almost stopped trying. Then Mark wisely took the initiative to prod me each and every night to lie in his arms whether I wanted to or not. After about two weeks of repeating this behavior without fail, I was amazed how desperately I wanted to fall asleep lying in his arms, and I looked forward to it all day. I was astonished to find my negative feelings were replaced gradually with positive feelings toward him and toward caring for him. I felt close to him again. It is a technique I recommend to everyone feeling separated from their spouse mentally or emotionally. Or try to come up with your own bed time activity or ritual.

I feel so grateful to have Mark in my life. I would rather have him and the MS than never to have had him at all. Not all days are fun. Not all nights are full of good cheer. Sometimes we get into ruts or fail to be inspired to go out and try new things. We are fortunate to have each other and fortunate that we discovered how fun bed can be. Why don't you get a room and try for yourself.

Anita Stienstra's work is published in *Prism Quarterly, Black Creek Review, Alchemist Review, Post Mortem Musings, Illinois Times, Chatham Clarion,* among others outlets. She is editor of *Navigating the Maze* and *Adonis Designs Press.* She has written for a weekly newspaper and taught writing and literature at two colleges. Born in Cleveland and raised near Valley Forge, she was educated at DePauw University and the University of Illinois at Springfield, and now lives near Lincoln's Home and Presidential Museum and Library.

Cute Shoes

Karen Fisher-Alaniz

"What happened to your head?" the secretary at my son's school asked.

"I ran into a brick wall," I said casually.

She stared.

"No really. I ran into a brick wall," I repeated. Suddenly I wanted to cry. I'd already laughed. I'd already looked at the bright side and the, *well it could have been worse* side. Now I wanted to cry.

Earlier that morning, I was running late for my physical therapy appointment. I was never late; I prided myself on that. But today I was. Today was my son's 5th grade graduation—I couldn't miss it! I'd had to miss so many other milestones. So I parked my car and hurried across the parking lot. I was on the sidewalk, just a few yards from the door of the building when it happened. One minute I was rushing to my appointment and the next I was lying on the sidewalk, bleeding. I tripped, I guess. I mean, the sidewalk was clear. There wasn't anything there to trip over. But nevertheless, I tripped. I found myself doing that oh-so-graceful slow motion, swimming through the air thing. But somehow, mid-fall, I had a millisecond of clarity: my misfortune didn't have to end in a sprawling face-plant on the sidewalk. I could catch myself on the side of the building, which was coming at me quickly. So in that moment I made a decision; I put my hands out in a bracing position and waited for the impact. But apparently I'd built up more momentum than I realized.

My hands hit the wall. Did I mention it was a brick wall? Yes. My hands hit the wall, and then, in one quick jerk, so did my head. In fact, I hit that wall so hard that I was thrown backwards, landing on my side a few feet away.

I lay there for a few seconds, afraid to move. This wasn't the first time I'd fallen, but it was the first time that I hoped and prayed someone had seen me. Then I heard a voice.

"Oh my gosh! Are you okay?" she yelled across the parking lot. I could hear shoes clicking toward me.

"Are you okay?" She asked again, kneeling beside me.

As I sat up, she looked me over, quickly surveying the damage. Both of my palms were cut, and my fingertips were cut too, nails sawed off jaggedly. My elbow had a huge gash in it, where I hit the sidewalk behind me.

"Oh," she said knowingly. "It was the shoes."

Several feet behind me were the cutest sandals you've ever seen. They were dark brown leather with tiny cream and turquoise beads sewn into a design of flowers and swirls. Cute, I'm telling you. They were so cute.

"You tripped over your shoes," she said. I said nothing. I kept quiet.

She opened the door for me and the usually serene place came alive. Nurses and receptionists surrounded me, doing what they could to comfort and care for me. I sat in a chair while they looked for Band-Aids for the tips of my fingers and gauze for the deep cuts on my hands. It was all pretty bad, but the worst was my elbow, which was dripping blood onto my jeans. I've got to get out of here, I thought. I didn't want to be rude, but my son was expecting me to be at his school in less than 45 minutes.

"That elbow's going to need stitches," one nurse said to the other. Then I remembered something else.

"I think I hit my head," I said. It was starting to throb. One of the nurses pulled my bangs back and her eyes got big.

"You sure did," she said. "You've got quite a goose egg here, and some scratches. What did you say you hit your head on?" As she gently applied an ice pack, I tried to explain.

"I really have to go," I said as they were finishing up.

"Is there someone we can call to pick you up?" she asked.

"No, thank you. I'm fine."

"I don't know.... That's quite a bump on your head."

"Really, I'm fine," I lied. My head was now pounding, but all I could think about was my son's 5th grade graduation. I couldn't miss this. Not this.

Fifteen minutes later, I was sitting in the gymnasium with all the other parents. I propped my camera between the scrapes on my hands and snapped pictures of my son singing, acting goofy with friends, and throwing his graduation cap. I was on my way out when the secretary caught me, asking about my head. I had no answer for her. No good answer anyway. And with tears threatening to explode I didn't want to stay and have some kind of public breakdown. I preferred to have my breakdowns in private.

After opening the car door with my uninjured thumb, I slid carefully into the driver's seat and drove home with my elbow held precariously in the air. Tears started to well. The adrenalin that had pumped through my veins after the fall had dissipated as the bandages were applied. Focusing on getting to my son's graduation had enabled me to not only get there, but even to enjoy the memorable event. My brain told me I should just go home and relax. But then there were the tears.

Once home, I stood barefoot, studying myself in the bathroom mirror. I used my thumb to pull my bangs back and laughed aloud when I saw the huge bump protruding from my forehead. Around it were scratches that looked suspiciously like the edges of bricks. Laughter gave way to tears as I replayed the five years since I'd been diagnosed.

Multiple sclerosis moved in without my permission. I'd only allowed it to stay because it refused to leave. It brought sinister housewarming gifts; muscles that tightened into painful spasms, mind-blurring fatigue and weakness, and most recently, memory problems. It had stolen from me, mocked me and taunted me. And now this.

Attending my son's graduation wasn't just about that one event. It was about all of the milestones I'd missed. It was about missing his first basketball game and the Easter egg hunt when he was six. It was about all of the changes I'd made to accommodate this disease.

"It was the shoes," the nurse had said. No it wasn't! I wanted to scream. It was this damn disease. I trip and fall all the time. I lose my balance and try not to lose my dignity along with it.

The time had come for me to give in to reality and wear more practical shoes. The doctor said so. My family said so. My friends said so. If it had been a real choice, that would be one thing. But it wasn't. "Haven't I lost enough?" I asked myself, looking in the mirror. "Can't I keep just this? Can't I keep my cute, color coor-dinated and completely impractical shoes?" Suddenly anger took over. I saw it in the mirror. The tears stopped and now I was fight-ing mad. I wanted to take MS and beat it to a pulp. I wanted to chuck it against a wall. I wanted to throw it to the ground and stomp on it.

A few days passed and then a few weeks. Those super-cute flip-flops were shuffled to the back of the closet and my wounds were healing.

"You should just throw them out," my husband said one day as I held them longingly.

"But I might wear them again."

"Karen," he said in his lecture tone that reminded me of my father, "I can't believe you didn't learn your lesson."

"I did," I said. "The next time I wear them, I'll be sure I have someone to hold on to. Like you."

Just as my son's graduation wasn't just about that one event, those flip-flops are not just about a pair of summer shoes. They are a symbol. Yes, there is grief tied up in them. But there is also hope. And there is determination. Those shoes might sit in my closet for ten more years. To some people that may seem silly, even ridiculous. But to me, keeping those shoes means MS has not won. It means that I didn't give up fighting and hoping. It means that although MS may be *in* me, it does not define who I am.

> "Keeping those shoes means MS has not won. It means that I didn't give up fighting and hoping."

I was at the shoe store the other day. I was surprised to see rows and rows of Converse sneakers, the kind I wore when I was much younger; when my body and I were still friends. There were low-tops and high tops. There were solids of every color imaginable and patterns of all kinds too.

I cringed as I conceded to the practicality of the shoes; they cover the whole foot, have non-skid soles and tie snuggly around the ankles.

"Converse are really coming back," the peppy little salesgirl said.

"There are so many colors," I answered, "I'd have to get a pair to match each of my different outfits. And that's *completely* impractical."

A smile crept across my face.

The peppy salesgirl looked confused as I left the store, a shiny bag dangling from my wrist.

"I'll be back," I said with confidence. "I will be back!"

Karen Fisher-Alaniz taught special education for fifteen years. When her disability progressed, she was forced to leave her job and begin a new chapter of her life. She is now writing full time. Her current project is writing her father's story of being a code breaker during World War Two. She lives in Washington State with her husband, Ric and her three children.

An Uplifting Exercise
Vicki L. Julian

It's easy to become disheartened or even depressed when multiple sclerosis rears its ugly head. But a simple desire to help someone facing a diagnosis enabled me to stumble upon an exercise to address these negative feelings. Before I retired on disability because of my own MS, a subordinate came to me in a fragile state. She had just learned that she might have MS, too, and since she knew of my condition, she was hoping for some encouragement. My first response was to tell her that my increasing dependence on a scooter for mobility was not a harbinger of what she might expect for herself if her diagnosis proved correct. I tried to help her understand that MS affects everyone differently, and that there was no way to determine the course of the disease. The point was simply, *"Don't use me or anyone else as an example!"*

Later that evening, while discussing with my husband my encounter with this young lady, it occurred to me what I could do for her, for myself and perhaps others as well. I decided to list everything that I had done in my life, beginning at what I now know was the first exacerbation, 29 years ago, divided into accomplishments before and after diagnosis. It was quite an eye-opener.

Surprisingly, mobility and fatigue issues aside, there wasn't really a difference in my successes pre- and post-diagnosis. I went on great vacations before and after diagnosis. I enjoyed physical challenges, such as parasailing, kayaking, and hiking before and after. I spent long hours at work before and after. I changed jobs before and after. I held highly responsible corporate positions before and after. I was involved in my church and community events before and after. I even had a child after my first undiagnosed exacerbation. While I had to give up some things, like dancing, surviving on little sleep to attend fun nights out, and taking long walks, I learned to compensate for these losses by focusing on what I still had and could do. I still loved and had the love of my family. I still hosted family events, and I still participated in the things that really mattered to me.

> "Concentrating on what you have done and are still doing helps keep you focused on the future."

While I have had more physical challenges in the two years since this initial exercise, I continue to add to my accomplishments. In short, the quality of my life hasn't changed since MS entered my life. And it was because of the list that I now realize it.

I recommend this exercise to all who have MS or, for that matter, anyone with a chronic illness, regardless of how your life has changed or how the disease has progressed. Some will note little difference, as I did, while others may see significant changes. But concentrating on what you have done and are still doing helps keep you focused on the future. For most of us, it puts the negatives into proper perspective. Just call it a lesson from Life 101.

Vicki Julian is the author of many business-themed works and has recently branched out into fiction writing. She published her first book in 2008. Vicki was diagnosed with MS in 1996 and is a peer advocate for the Teva Neuroscience-sponsored Shared Solutions program.

Part IV
The MS Family

Recollection
Rachel E. Pollock

I can't recall if I ever saw my mother dance.

Our relationship was never what you might call "sporty." It was my father who tossed a ball with me in the yard, my father who showed me how to build snowmen and took me on long bike rides through quiet small-town streets. It was he who taught me the cannonball and the sailor's dive while my mother smiled poolside beneath a sunhat, behind a book. But if my father was a snowball fight and that first shaky ride without training wheels, my mother was a warm cup of cocoa and a Band-Aid for my skinned knee.

I try to remember, what might we have done before her diagnosis, before the beautifully-spiraling Lucite cane, before the wheeled walker or the electric scooter or the ever-changing parade of pills and injections. What had we then that is now lost? What might I miss—what might she—that is now forever denied, impossible?

Throughout my childhood we traveled a lot as a family. That hasn't changed. She and my father still go on yearly vacations—whatever strikes their fancy, whether it be Broadway plays or driving tours of the national parks—and though I am in my thirties now, sometimes I still go along, too. She and my dad book their trips much as they always did, though now she ferrets out handicap-accessible accommodations; he packs the battery charger for her ultra-lightweight compactable scooter, and off they go. She'll even joke about the perks of traveling with the disabled: "First ones on the plane, front row seats in the theatre, and all the best parking places reserved!" No, she'll never climb Macchu Picchu now, but I'm not sure she would have before the MS anyway.

Her career has changed drastically since she was first diagnosed. She was a lawyer back then, in those carefree ambulant days—one of the first female lawyers to practice in our tiny Southern town. As a girl, I didn't understand the ethical nuances of a law career, but she and her few women colleagues were pioneer role models to me, beautiful but dangerous with their softly rolled hairstyles and smart case-trying suits. But it wasn't MS that led her to abandon the courts in favor of a professorship at the local state university. "Frankly, being a lawyer was boring," she'll say if you ask her about it. "Teaching, now that's exciting!"

Many things, though, are quite the same: Charles Dickens is still her favorite author; Chanel No. 5 is still her favorite perfume. She loves live theatre, Mexican food, lowbrow humor, classical music, house-cat antics, the smell of pine sap, Caravaggio paintings, raspberry crepes as a late breakfast, Patrick O'Brien novels read aloud, cheap white wine in champagne flutes, scratchy-voiced country singers, and staying up till 2 A.M. talking about a thousand different things in front of a winter hearth—these things have not changed.

Walking around in the fields of memory, I can't find a recollection of her just standing alone, unsupported, her hand not outstretched toward something that's caught her eye, not resting on a banister nor clasped within my father's or my own. I remember us in shopping centers and museums and I think, she must have been walking on her own, mustn't she? We still go together to those places, to malls and art galleries and archaeology exhibits; I might have coltishly outstripped her as a girl, running ahead while she lagged behind, but with her scooter she moves faster than I do now.

I know MS is a trial for her, a continual challenge that weaves its insidious threads through even the most mundane fabric of her day. Her struggles don't pass beneath my notice—the waning dexterity, the balance and stamina losses, her hypersensitivity to climate change, the slightest of which may affect her coordination. I see her always striving to do more, to push herself—don't stop driving a car, don't stop writing by hand, cook Christmas dinner no matter what (even though now Dad handles the batter-mixing and the potato-mashing and the putting of casseroles into the oven, and I take care of the tablecloths and place settings and pouring of drinks). I admire the strength that allows her to push against the MS, to be so much more than a diagnosis, more than "just" a disabled person, to retain every scrap of herself in the face of it.

> "No, she'll never climb Macchu Picchu now, but I'm not sure she would have before the MS anyway."

I'd be lying if I said it didn't affect how I see her and think of her—that strength and determination and bravery color my perception, certainly, but the harsh light of her condition reveals her as a woman whose character is that to which I can only aspire. It is her weakness that brings out her strength, and I think that, because I have always thought of her as a strong and capable person, this is why I have difficulty remembering her as someone who once could do something that now she cannot. I can't remember her walking or running, jumping or dancing, perhaps because who she is in my heart transcends any physical form or ability.

Certainly, I wish she were healthy and whole. Certainly, I know that once she must have danced—at her high school prom, with my grandfather at her wedding reception, perhaps even in triumph after sending my croquet ball flying out of wicket-range, though I cannot now recollect.

No, when I remember my mother before she had MS, she is never standing alone in those memories. Then, as now, her hand is firmly clasped in my father's or in mine, sometimes for support, but always, foremost, with love.

———————

Rachel E. Pollock is a professional theatre and film costumer and lecturer for the graduate program in Costume Production at the University of North Carolina at Chapel Hill. Her writing has appeared in a *Southern Arts Journal, Harvard Summer Review*, the anthology *Knoxville Bound* and elsewhere. Her mother, Eugenea C. Pollock, was diagnosed with multiple sclerosis over twenty years ago and continues to teach a full course load at the College of Business at East Tennessee State University.

The Good, the Bad and the Ugly
Beth Shaw

The Good

Craig and I met while serving on the same ship in the Navy. We were married within a year, I left the Navy, and we had two unexpected but absolutely wonderful children. The first few years were great. We struggled for money at times, but we were a happy family. Craig stayed in the Navy, hoping to finish his 20 years and retire, and I worked my way up from server to manager at Applebee's. During these years we took the kids to the beach whenever we could, got together with friends to play cards or grill out, went down to the waterfront for Friday night concerts in the park; it seemed as if we were always going somewhere and having fun. Then one day I was called to the Naval Hospital at Norfolk. Something had happened to Craig.

The Bad

No one at the hospital knew for sure what was happening. I was told Craig could have hit his head and suffered a concussion; I was told he may have suffered a stroke. I was devastated. They wouldn't let me see him and I had no family in Norfolk. I was lost, worried, and confused, and could only imagine what he was going through. I was relieved when I was finally allowed to see him, but that relief was short-lived when I saw that he could barely move to hug me and his words were so slurred I couldn't understand what he was trying to say. The doctors had, by this time, ruled out stroke and described his condition as serious but stable. Craig underwent several more tests throughout the course of the day while his symptoms began to subside. The doctors still had no idea what had caused his symptoms or why they had to come and gone so quickly, but they said there was no reason to keep him any longer. We made an appointment with a neurologist and we went home.

Over the course of the next few months he had flare ups of these same symptoms, although none were as severe as on the day he was taken to the E.R. He saw the neurologist, several times in fact, and he ran just about every test he could on Craig, including a spinal tap and several M.R.I.s. We saw this neurologist for over a year before we finally got a diagnosis: Relapsing-Remitting Primary Progressive Multiple Sclerosis. I don't remember all the details of what we did next; we were both in a daze.

Craig knew more than the average bear when it came to MS because his older sister has it, but I knew almost zero. I went to the library and picked up just about every book I could find on MS. Between the brochures I'd taken from the doctor's office and the books from the library I was up all night trying to learn as much as I could. I was afraid to talk with Craig's sister about it. In fact, I tried to block out the fact that she even had it. She was still in her 30s and already wheelchair-bound. I was nowhere near ready to face the thought that my beloved husband might suffer the same fate.

So, we learned what we could about the disease. Craig did his best to cope with the erratic symptoms and I did my best to help him. Sometimes we talked about it, sometimes we got mad about it, many times we just held each other, and life went on.

About two years after his diagnosis, Craig had an attack that landed him in the hospital on intravenous steroids for five days.

He lost the sight in his right eye and it has never come back. Eventually, the Navy allowed him to retire with full benefits after 19 years of service. We decided to move close to my family, in case we needed help. I didn't admit it, but I remembered how awful, how lonely, I felt during that first visit to the E.R. and I never again wanted to go through an experience like that alone.

So we moved to a small town in Kentucky and went about our lives. I was still managing Applebee's and Craig pretty much was Mr. Mom. He continued (and still continues) to have flare ups. Occasionally he required steroids but those were administered by home healthcare rather than at the hospital. Considering how sick he was and could be again at the drop of a hat, we felt pretty lucky. We certainly didn't let the disease control our lives. Much of the time it was like it wasn't even there.

The Ugly

Seven years after Craig retired and ten years since his diagnoses, I got sick. Within six months, I was diagnosed with rheumatoid arthritis, fibromyalgia, and hypothyroidism. My arthritis was so severe and progressive that I was soon forced to quit work and file for disability benefits. Within nine months of my diagnosis, I was wheelchair-bound. Craig and I were back on that roller-coaster of emotions we first rode when he was diagnosed. But by this time, our kids were old enough to help out around the house and Craig, while still experiencing sometimes severe symptoms, was at least able to stay out of the hospital and remain capable of walking.

> "Life is so random and coincidental that sometimes we just have to laugh about it."

Life is so random and coincidental that sometimes we just have to laugh about it. I mean, here two healthy young people meet, marry, have kids, and they both end up with autoimmune diseases with very similar symptoms and with absolutely no way to predict when any or all of these symptoms might flare up. We've each, together and alone, thought we couldn't take it anymore. But what are you going to do? We have two kids, family who love us, and perhaps most importantly, we have each other. This brings me to:

Just Don't Forget the Hope

> *"I wept because I had no shoes,*
> *until I saw a man who had no feet."*
>
> *Persian proverb*

For people like us who are dealing with diseases like Craig's MS, this is the point at which folks you're talking with say things like, "...there are new medical advances every day..." or, "I just read this article about a new..." I could go on and on, but you get the idea. They mean well, but Craig and I found that if you are relying on them—or *anyone else* besides yourself—to keep your hope alive, then it will surely die. In one way, Craig and I are lucky: we both have similar autoimmune diseases and we can talk to each other without sympathy or pity. But even he and I have to keep looking *inside*.

The hope I am talking about is the kind that keeps us going mentally; the kind that sees to it we get up every morning, brush our teeth, comb our hair, and get dressed whether we plan to leave the house that day or not. Maybe hope is the wrong word, but I can't think of a better one to describe why we choose to continue to actively live our lives and be involved in the lives of those we love. Craig and I have found many things to hope for; here are just a few:

Health and happiness for our children.

To be able to enjoy our future grandchildren.

That maybe telling about some of our medical and health-related experiences can help someone else.

Better health and fewer flare ups for Craig.

That our children have a much easier adulthood than they did childhoods. They deserve it.

That we will never forget all we have to be grateful for.

That we will never allow ourselves to lose hope.

The list could go on and on, and we can't help but think that it's the hard times that have made these hopes so clear to us, and we're thankful for that.

Beth Shaw was born in Cape Girardeau, Missouri and resided in Owensboro, Kentucky until she passed away unexpectedly on October 6th, 2007. She is sorely missed by her children and her husband, Craig.

Memories of Home
Myrna Beth Lambert

My husband Larry and I bought this house 35 years ago because we loved how its rooms flow from floor to floor, staircase to staircase. There are stairs everywhere in this house.

It is a large home filled with memories of our family. The double front door opens into a long foyer that leads into the family room with its brick fireplace and sliding doors. In this room we roasted marshmallows by the fireplace and hung stockings from the mantel on Christmas Eve. Through the sliding doors we can view the spacious yard that once held swings, a slide and a sandbox. Today I look through the glass doors and my memory plays tricks. For a fleeting moment I see my little girls playing outdoors and I can hear their laughter as they swing to the moon or try to touch the stars.

To reach the next level of our home, the dining room and kitchen area, one must walk up three stairs. We have held multitudes of family dinners in these two rooms. The dining room echoes with the joy of our family gatherings. Three steps down from the dining room is the living room. In this room I visualize our daughters seated at the piano playing their favorite songs and practicing for their recitals.

It's a climb of nine steps from the dining room to reach the bedrooms. Standing at the top of these stairs I can still hear our children's laughter, their tears and their fights. I hear their lengthy telephone conversations with friends as the sounds of music from their tape decks wrap around the walls. In this house we held our daughters' birthday parties and entertained their friends. In wintertime, Larry would take the three little girls sledding on the hill behind the house and he taught them to swim in the heat of summer in our back yard. The pool was my husband's one luxurious indulgence for himself and his family.

> "The reasons we loved this house are the reasons we must leave it."

We loved this house when we purchased it and have loved it ever since. Perhaps we love it most on this day. Because, sadly, the reasons we loved this house are the reasons we must leave it: Larry has multiple sclerosis and can barely walk. In recent years our home's many stairs have become mountains for him. We have tried to alter the house to accommodate his needs, but even with a chair lift and a motorized scooter upstairs he is still unable to get around. This house was not built for a disabled person, and all the modifying we have done does not make the house any more accessible for my husband. We have stretched our time spent here to the limit. Each year we have said that next year we must move before we run out of time. Now we have. Sometimes Larry can't get downstairs because the short walk from the bedroom to the chair lift feels like miles to him. His lovely house is becoming his prison, and this beautiful home was never meant to impart such negative vibes. But all those positive reasons we had for loving our house are the reasons we now have for disliking it. So we must move on.

It is hard to say goodbye to the home we have shared most of our married life. When I look at my disabled husband, I still see the handsome young man who took on the responsibilities of husband, father and homeowner with all the maturity of a man twice his age. Now, this morning, I can see my handsome young lawyer in his pinstripe suit going off to work through the same double front door we will soon pass through for the last time. This has been the family home for more than our generation: our children have married and bring our grandchildren here to visit. They swim in the pool and play in the playroom, creating for us a second vision of our youth. But the joys of entertaining our grandchildren can not compensate for the confinement Larry experiences living within these walls. I must keep reminding myself that the grandchildren will visit wherever we dwell. That these memories will not end when we close that door behind us.

The movers are approaching. It is time to say farewell to our home. But the memories are etched within my heart. I shall take them with me and store them in a place where I can retrieve them when I get lonely for our first home. We are at a different place in life than we were 35 years ago and we must begin to accumulate new memories. One is never too old for new beginnings.

Myrna Beth (Micki) Lambert is the mother of three grown daughters and eight grandchildren. She has been married to her husband Stan for forty years. Micki writes poetry and short stories and has had several poems and stories published locally. She divides her time between homes in Chicago and Florida.

The Trapeze Diaries
Marie Carter

The aerialist caught the hoop beautifully every time, some-times with her feet, sometimes with her arms, sometimes with her ankles, once with her head. She projected long shad-ows against the wall of the tent. Many times I thought she might fall and break her neck, but she didn't. It was the first time I'd seen anything like it. From a distance, she looked perfect. She did not seem to sweat. She did not seem to breathe. Her body appeared weightless. She was so far above me she could have been an angel.

Later, I couldn't stop thinking about her. I was so touched by the way she defied everything human in herself: unafraid of heights, flexible and strong. That night, I dreamt shadows were dancing above me. I thought I was falling from a trapeze and I woke to my own shuddering.

When I was 22, my father died of a sudden heart attack. He had died at a point in my life that was a flurry of activity. I had exams to pass, money to earn; I was in the process of moving from Scotland to New York; I had packing to do and an internship to complete. I was determined not to cry in front of anyone, my mother included. I wanted to appear strong. I didn't want grief to take up my time. Most of all, I didn't want to upset my mother who had been threatening, "If your father goes, I go." She kept saying it so decidedly, my brother and I believed her.

Several months after my father's death, I graduated from college and moved to New York. Then the grief and sadness mounted. Sometimes on the subway I'd cry for no apparent reason while people looked the other way. I never realized that grief could last so long.

On her first visit to New York, my mother asked, "Do you ever think about your dad?" and I wanted to tell her, "All the time," but I didn't.

After I saw the aerialist perform I bought souvenirs: a CD, a T-shirt and a pen, but when I got home realized it wasn't enough. There was something else I wanted, something not quite tangible that I had left behind. And for weeks after the circus I walked around with this feeling.

During my lunch breaks, in the summer, I have been walking to the Westside Highway to watch people taking lessons at the flying trapeze school. I feel envious as strong, flexible men and women fly through the air and hang upside down by their knees. Then they roll off the net, faces red with exhilaration.

My friend Christa was a gymnast, starting at the age of six. She gave it up as a teenager because she was so good at it that the other kids hated her for running off with all the trophies. I tell her I'd been thinking about studying trapeze. She urges me to do so while I'm still young. She's now in her forties.

Shortly after her first visit to New York, my mother was diagnosed with multiple sclerosis. Her symptoms had become most pronounced after my father's death. She would often lose her balance and have difficulty walking. For the year before she was diagnosed, the doctor, telling her it was "just grief," had been prescribing anti-depressants and sleeping pills. The hospital staff were continually setting her up with appointments for scans, then sending her for the wrong ones.

When my mother first learned she had MS she was full of fear, saying things like, "I could go blind," or "Next year I could be in a wheelchair."

Every time I have to meet her on a street corner, I worry even if she is only five minutes late. I imagine her passed out on the sidewalk somewhere or falling on the subway stairs. But she always turns up, smiling.

There is a poster for a missing old lady in the window of the pastry shop near where I live. I wonder where in New York one might find a missing old lady.

"Your father wasn't very patient with illness," my mother says. "He didn't like it when I was ill. He'd get cross and tell me I was imagining things."

I started looking at my own body for signs of decay. MS can be inherited. Sometimes I would imagine little pockets of foreign bodies lying dormant in my organs, ready to awaken and destroy me.

"Circus people make this look so damn easy," the aerialist says, pointing at the trapeze. I have taken Christa's advice and signed up for my first trapeze lesson. "But it takes so much patience and it hurts like hell. You're probably going to cry; you'll get angry and frustrated. You'll definitely bruise and most likely you'll get scared. Obviously we don't want any serious injuries, but it's good for you to challenge yourself. Let fear teach you; it's good to have a healthy amount of fear."

When she visited New York, my mother found it hard to walk and had to be met at the airport with a wheelchair. I couldn't stand the thought of leaving my home in New York and going back to Scotland, yet I felt enormous guilt about not being there for her. Every time she leaves New York, I think this will be the last time I'll see her. Sometimes I panic and have difficulty breathing. I spend the last few days of her visit crying, and can't seem to stop, even when I'm at work. I am so embarrassed I have to keep running to the bathroom to calm down.

The aerialist decides we should work on Bird's Nest, one of the simplest tricks. I take my turn: Upside down, my hands holding the bar and my knees hooked over it, I slide my legs up the rope then curl and arch my back, turning under to face the other side of the room, hanging from the bar as if about to dive into a pool. This seems like it should be easy to do, but it takes several tries for me to get it, and other students are watching, so I have a hard time focusing on the movement. I feel embarrassed, scared and self-conscious. This was a stupid idea, I tell myself, since I'm scared of heights and of being upside down.

The woman taking her turn after me nails Bird's Nest on her first try. She is destined to be a trapeze artist; I am not. I have my doubts that I can get good at trapeze. I'm stuck in the memory of the past when I was a high school girl and always the last in school races or the last to get picked for hockey teams. To myself I admit my resemblance to my mother—I am more faithful to the story of the past than to the one unfolding in front of me.

The aerialist says, "Watch out for those negative thoughts. If you keep telling yourself you can't do something, your body will give you exactly what you want."

While on vacation in New Mexico, I meet a psychic.

"You're worried about someone," she says, revealing the obvious. I tell her about my mother who is suffering from MS.

"That's an auto-immune disease. It's the body attacking itself. You say that she was diagnosed shortly after your father died. She's subconsciously trying to kill herself."

I change the subject. Part of me is offended that she would say such a thing about my mother but she has also addressed a long-held fear of mine—I've always worried that my mother has been trying to kill herself off and that I'd lose her suddenly the way I lost my dad. She often points out that my Uncle John died of a heart attack several months after his wife died.

"He died of a broken heart," she said.

When my mother takes up smoking, I scold her. When she talks to me on the phone I can hear the long exhalations of cigarette smoke.

"Don't talk to me while you're smoking," I say, both angry and frightened. Is she trying to destroy herself?

Whenever my mother used to send me things from Scotland, I could always smell home on the packages. Now they smell of home and cigarette smoke.

The aerialist makes me try Bird's Nest again but the trick feels impossible.

"You need to be okay with where you're at," the aerialist says. "You know some people would be ecstatic if they could just touch their toes."

My mother and I are walking through Central Park where people are rollerblading, biking and running. My mother has to walk very slowly and take breaks on a park bench every fifteen minutes. She tells me not to take my young body for granted. "I used to study yoga in my thirties and I could do a full lotus in headstand."

It is distressing for me to see how much she has declined. While her body has been deteriorating, I have been getting stronger. "It's amazing

"It's good to have a healthy amount of fear."

what other people can do with their bodies," she says. "When I was first struck with multiple sclerosis and I had trouble walking, I used to get so envious and frustrated. But now I've come to accept my limitations and I'm working with the illness."

My mother is full of the belief that I am going to do very well in life. And when I do become rich and famous, I'll buy her a holiday home in a hot country like France and take her sailing on my personal yacht.

"It may not happen for another ten or twenty years," she says. "I may even be eighty by the time you become rich and famous, but that's okay because I can wait until then."

I feel relieved: my mother has promised to live until she's eighty.

Marie Carter moved from Edinburgh, Scotland to Brooklyn, New York in 2000. She has had work published in *The Best Creative Nonfiction*, *Hanging Loose*, *Brooklyn Rail*, *Bloom*, turntablebluelight.com, and *Spectacle*, among others. She is the editor of *Word Jig: New Fiction from Scotland*. She completed a residency at the MacDowell Colony in 2006 and her book *The Trapeze Diaries* is forthcoming.

Multiple Memories
Raquelle Azran

A family legend tells that during the polio epidemic of the Fifties, which left thousands of children paralyzed, Mom negotiated with God. "Spare my three year-old daughter and take me instead," she bargained. I emerged unscathed from the epidemic, and she was diagnosed with MS. This reinforced her belief in an omnipotent God, a divine being for whom a deal is a deal.

Firstborn daughters of strong women are purported to be independent of spirit, precocious learners and verbally adept. I tend to believe that my mother, also a firstborn child, was all of the above. Her intellectual streak went hand in hand with fierce integrity. In an era of racism and discrimination, her colorblindness toward human beings was legendary. Had MS not begun doing its dirty work on her in the Sixties, I can see Mom espousing feminism with a passion.

Yet a deal was made, and deals must be kept. Mom's God demanded his due, and her legs were the first sacrifice. Sporadic attacks of sensation loss were followed by a gradual yet unremitting weakening. No more tennis, no more running, no more hikes. Even short walks now required several rest intervals. My earliest memories are of hearing Mom's apologetic "my stupid legs" whenever she needed to sit down.

But neither God nor chronic diseases are of interest to a little girl who wants a mother like everyone else's. I wanted someone who pops out to shop, jumps up to serve dinner, runs over to friends and is able to catch me when I run around the glass dinner table, escaping a no doubt justified slap. My mother could do none of the above. Mom became a weakly benevolent presence, full of good intentions and almost bursting with a desire to please absolutely everyone, a surefire recipe for self-annihilation if ever there was one. And since using a cane, crutches or wheelchair was admitting defeat, or reality, Mom nixed all those options and staggered unassisted from wall to table to chair, and there were many times she didn't make it and ended up on the floor.

Everyone in the family found a different way of coping with Mom's handicap. Her parents pretended it didn't exist. "Margot is tired today," they would remark during their visits, as Mom lunged at a wall. "Will you please stop trying to walk around," my Dad would grate as he roughly hauled her up from yet another sprawl. Bound by his sense of loyalty to my mother yet unable to summon up the endless reserves of empathy which could perhaps have substituted for love, my father immersed himself in his business. Four days a week, every week, were spent out of town. And because his demands on my mother were so minimal, she tried even harder to please him. Wearing just a nightgown under her coat in the early morning chill, slippers sliding dangerously on the frosty driveway, Mom would drive Dad out to the airport. His favorite dinner of vegetable soup and fish would be awaiting his return, along with tremulous embraces.

> "Unable to face the relentless deterioration in her condition, I was anywhere my mother wasn't."

And where was I all those years? Unable to face the relentless deterioration in her condition, I was anywhere my mother wasn't. I searched endlessly for surrogate mothers among my teachers and my friends' mothers, spending as little time at home as possible. From school I continued straight to the public library, and when it closed at six I made the rounds of my friends, seeking out dinner invitations. I was the first kid to beg to sleep over at friends' homes, and go away to relatives for the weekend.

But it was not only my mother's physical presence I evaded. Figuratively as well, I consciously negated my mother. To me, she signified failure, weakness, an inability to cope. She played bridge—I avoided it. She listened only to classical music—I cranked up the volume of Grace Slick and The Doors. She found dressing up and makeup a waste of time—I spent endless hours on the finer points of miniskirts, skintight jeans and false eyelashes.

Meanwhile, MS was busily expanding its conquest. Mom's kidneys were the next victim. In addition to always being on the lookout for elevators and ramps, Mom now had to worry about having a bathroom available, immediately. The MPH on road signs, we cruelly decided, meant "Mom peed here." Now I had a mother who was not only handicapped but also incontinent. I left home. Correction—I fled, as far away as I could. I escaped to study overseas.

Safely separated by an ocean, my mother and I became penpals. In handwriting steadily deteriorating as the MS invaded her arms, she wrote of her daily activities and inquired about mine. Over the years, I outgrew my adolescent desire to shock her and wrote comforting tales of family, children and career. I wrote her that now I, too, enjoyed classical music, and that my oldest daughter inherited her penchant for bridge. I teased her that her hopes for "an intellectual housewife of a daughter" (a wish she had expressed to a reporter while wheeling me in my baby carriage, memorialized in a yellowed newspaper clipping) had even then been hopelessly passe.

She gently stung back by reminding me that she had studied for her doctorate at the age of 19, and when was I ever going to make time in my busy schedule for a doctorate, let alone a husband.

My mother's scrawl eventually grew indecipherable to everyone except me. I awaited with dread her weekly letters detailing how the MS invaded her eyes and mind. She shared with me the horrors of seeing giant spiders on the walls, knowing she was hallucinating, yet unable to quell the terror. She wrote of accusing my father of trying to remove her wedding ring before murdering her, of realizing it was a nightmare, but still being paralyzed with fear. Often I left her letters unopened for a day or two, hoping they would be mislaid and I would then be spared the reading. Unfortunately, one cannot flee reality as easily at thirty-five as at sixteen years of age.

After almost three decades of disease, the MS struck again, this time fatally. Urgently summoned home when Mom's condition became critical, I entered my mother's room, expecting to find her unconscious or at least confused. She smiled up at me, turned to my father and said, "Martin, look who's here to visit. It's my daughter, my very best friend."

A native New Yorker, Raquelle Azran divides her time between Hanoi, Vietnam, where she specializes in Vietnamese contemporary fine art and Tel Aviv, Israel, where she writes in her inner city aerie overlooking the Mediterranean.

The Suction Tube

Marion Deutsche Cohen

For ten years Jeff had a suction tube by his bed in Inglis House. At first he'd mutter his usual brand of denial: "I don't really need it. It's just for security." Later he stopped saying that; it was obvious that he did need it, more and more frequently.

"Asking for it" meant asking me to take it off the hook, put it in his mouth—just close enough to his throat to get at what needed to be suctioned out, but not close enough to choke him. Little bits of brownery and greenery floated down that transparent tube. It collected in a transparent cylinder, a slimy ocean to imagine bathing in.

In other words, yuck.

Ah, but it was so great to not be doing nights, lifting, and toilet. It felt almost wonderful to simply watch the aides do all that. It required three or more at a time, whereas just a few months before, when he lived at home, I had done it by myself. I didn't exactly gloat as I watched the aides but I did feel extremely grateful.

Nights for me now were a high as well as a relief. I could barely believe that an entire night would pass, again and again, without me being awakened by his voice, a cross between demanding and plaintive. "Mar, couldja hand me a jar." "Handing him a jar" had involved also holding it for him, sometimes for fifteen minutes or so, because "incontinent" doesn't only mean not knowing when you have to go; it also means taking a long time to go, or not finishing and then needing to go again. "Handing him a jar" had also included waiting until I could take off the jar, then traipsing to the bathroom to clean it, then putting it back for when he'd need it again, often within another hour.

That this didn't happen anymore was, for me, literally a miracle. And for him? Well, for him it did happen, but now "it" was a catheter. He didn't like them especially, but the aides at Inglis House couldn't and wouldn't hand him a jar every hour or every fifteen minutes during the night. There would be no miracles, literal or otherwise, for him.

"I hope that, when you're ready, you'll start dating," suggested a friend. Another friend, my best friend actually, surprised me one day and asked, "Do you have a lover?" The answer to the first friend was, I wasn't ready. And to the second, "Of course not. I'd tell you right away if I was."

One reason that I wasn't ready was that I still loved my husband, in some ways, or I thought that I might. Another reason was that, not only had I had enough sex for awhile—in particular, enough "disability sex", enough of the kind of sex where I had to be the active one. What I needed, after six years of nights, lifting, and toilet, was to be the passive one, in a lot of ways. I needed to be taken care of—again, in a lot of ways. Treated, yes, like a child, and not like an adult, in particular, an adult sexual being.

Besides, I was scared.

He had a busy schedule at the nursing home. In nursing homes "busy work" is very important for the residents to have. And Inglis House kept us both busy. He and I made the rounds: P.T., O.T., ham radio club, shul, support group twice a week (called Friends on Wheels), meetings with doctors about things like what would go into the feeding tube. Sometimes the nursing home kept me busy in ways that I liked. I was asked to do poetry readings, first for Friends on Wheels then in their main auditorium. The residents said that it was helpful to them to hear what their relatives and caregivers were feeling. In general, it was kind of fun being an "Inglis House wife;" it was sort of like being a faculty wife or a "soccer mom."

My husband and I would hold hands at the Friends on Wheels meetings. Sometimes Devin, our eight year-old, would join us at the meetings. The other members of the group liked us, and welcomed those of us not on wheels as "honorary" members. In general, both Devin and I got into the "disability spirit." But my husband never seemed to be in that spirit, or in any spirit. He did have a kind of dry humor, to his very end, and that was appreciated by the staff, or at least reacted to. Basically, though, he just didn't feel happy. Often, when everyone else was smiling or laughing, I would catch sight of his very straight face.

One of the hardest things about visiting someone—anyone—in a nursing home or hospital is leaving. The person doesn't want you to go. And as soon as leaving time draws nigh, suddenly all sorts of things need to be done. The pillow needs adjusting, or the blow tube. Or one more suctioning. Or there's something he forgot to tell you. Or ask you. Or all of the above.

Towards the end of a visit was also around the time that an aide would knock on the door.

"Jeff, what time would you like to go to bed?"

"Six-thirty," Jeff would answer, "Because Marion's here."

He would forget that I always left at 5, to catch the bus and be home before dark.

It would get complicated, or feel complicated. Somehow it took me a while to get assertive and tell the aide what time I was actually leaving. Eventually I did.

But I couldn't bear to be assertive about the many objects at home that he remembered. "Do we still have that hospital bed?" "What about that physics book?" The hospital bed had been laboriously moved to the room opposite our bedroom at home. It was extremely large and turquoise blue. Its mattress was only half blown up and it looked pretty ridiculous. As for the physics books, there were many of them; his small room at the nursing home couldn't possibly accommodate them all. So if and when he needed such-and-such a book, he'd ask me to bring it.

The bedroom in which I now slept alone was also too small to accommodate all of his physics books, and I had zilch emotional attachment to them. But I couldn't bear, and didn't dare, to move too many of them, for fear of not being able to find them when Jeff asked for them. "I need to look up a formula in Whitaker and Watson," he'd tell me. "It's on the bottom shelf towards the right." Sometimes he was right and sometimes he wasn't. And sometimes he truly did need to look up that formula and sometimes he didn't. But even when it was crystal clear that he wasn't going to be coming home for any holidays, I didn't get anybody to cart that turquoise bed or those books down to the cellar.

And even as he lay on his deathbed I didn't completely clear out those bookcases. I was never certain that Jeff wouldn't need them and accuse me of having thrown or given them away.

I understood his need to have at least some of his things in his house: the house he never saw again once he entered the nursing home, the house he knew was no longer safe for him to be in for more than an hour or so because, for example, it contained no suction tube.

Often, sometimes two or three times in one week, he needed to go to the hospital because his J-tube would come dislodged. The nursing home wasn't equipped to take care of things like that. I would usually meet him at the emergency room, but if I happened to be visiting him at the time, I'd go along with him in the ambulance. I didn't particularly want to do any of it. It got to be a pain in the neck, and I needed to get home in time for the kids.

But it was sad. Jeff was scared. He didn't entirely trust the ambulance people, no matter how well trained they seemed and were. One characteristic of multiple sclerosis, in his case, was fear to the point of paranoia. It usually took precedence over any love for or consideration of me and the kids.

But sometimes it didn't. One time he kept saying, over and over again, "Thank you for coming along with me." Then, when the hospital dismissed him, he asked the ambulance people whether they could drive me back to my house. And when they couldn't, "Take a taxi," he told me seriously and significantly. We both remembered that one of our issues had been taxis, and other expensive things. He had wanted to save money, too often. In his better moments he now, too late, understood that. Or maybe he simply wanted to please me, for fear I'd stop visiting him. When the taxi and the ambulance both arrived at the same time, we went our separate ways. He to his home, me to mine.

> "But did I still love him? Should I have loved him?"

Some visits were good. I'd tell him about troubles and vulnerabilities at work and he'd say, "Don't worry, Mar, you're okay," and, "You're the best teacher, that's obvious." And it helped. But did I still love him? *Should* I have loved him? After all those nights, liftings, and toilets, after his denial of it all, his choice, conscious and subconscious, to look after himself rather than me and the kids. We still could, in his good moments, share his physics and my math. I could still, at least at times, turn to him for reassurance. Indeed, I still *knew* him, and he me. But, during those long years, was to know him to love him, like the song? One thing I was sure of, at least during those early nursing-home years: when he was gone I would miss him.

Many of the other residents also had sagging spirit, and expressionless faces. Why?

I sometimes wondered. They're not paralyzed above the neck. Faces were all they had left; why didn't they want to use them? Maybe, I answered myself, *people really don't like to use all they have left.*

Jeff's condition was also mental, there was no denying that. Decades ago, doctors used to believe that multiple sclerosis was "merely" neurological, but now they know that, in some cases, it's also mental. In some ways. And that's the problem. At first only the spouse notices it. Maybe some close, and wise, friends. It often doesn't affect the intellect; Jeff could still discuss physics and math and he still worked on papers. He could still remember names, numbers, and what happened both last week and fifty years ago. Or some of it. He could still swallow and chew. He could watch TV, getting the correct channels via the blow tube.

Sometimes the only thing dementia affects is judgment. In particular, financial judgment. And the health care system and its laws haven't caught up with that finding. It's into denial about that kind of dementia, meaning that it doesn't and can't legally declare people with it "incompetent." So family members of people with such "subtle" dementia are, eventually, caught in a lot of nightmare. Over the years that would happen to me and my kids.

But for now his fingers could still grip mine. I knew it was just a spasm but it still felt nice. And we could still bring him food from Tandoor India. But food to go is never as good as food actually eaten at the restaurant. Jeff wanted so badly for it to be like old times with the family together in Tandoor India, but it couldn't be. Not even close.

A year and a half after he went to live in the nursing home, Jeff's MS began to progress some more. Progression is gradual, they say, but in some sense it's gradual only as the years pass. If you're with it week by week, it often seems sudden. And all of a sudden I began to feel heartbroken for him. The progression showed in his voice. His chest. Often he could barely muster the air to get sound out. It was not difficult to communicate with him but I could feel the effort that he needed to put in. His speech was no longer a given. Sometimes I'd get into his bed with him and he would just whisper as we cuddled. He didn't seem to have trouble whispering, not then.

And his energy level seemed to be the same; he didn't usually feel tired. But he was scared and he sometimes admitted it. "Why did I get sick?" he'd ask, and "If I get completely better, what would you like to do?" We'd talk about thrift-shopping together, restaurants, maybe he'd join in making supper, and maybe he'd play Scrabble or some other game.

He was scared. Dinner time was when that showed up most. The aide was patient, and Jeff kept trying that patience. Kept asking, again and again, for his pillow to be adjusted; there seemed to be no true position for that pillow. And the bed—the head part, and the foot part too. And then, of course, the food itself. A little more of this, a lot more of that. Could that last spoonful be scooped up more thoroughly?

Leaving time was getting more and more poignant. "Too bad," he'd murmur, with a kind of dignified acceptance. The more scared he became, the more things he asked for. The more things around the room needed fixing, the more twisted became the respirator chin strap hanging on the pole, and the saggier became the blow tube. "I can't tell them what I need," he'd gasp, then, "Can you stretch my right arm again?"

He had more strength to whisper than we had to listen to him. "We" meant the aides, the kids, and I. We had to bend down, straining, put our ears first to the right, then to the left. And we had to be standing up. And to keep telling Devin shush.

Sometimes—more and more rarely—memories and old feelings emerged. Eating out in Chili's one evening with Devin, Jeff had been unusually pleasant to be with, attentive to Devin and careful not to obsess about the food. Best of all, when we had gotten back from Chili's and were settled in his room, I noticed that he had something wrapped up in a napkin lying on the chest. I knew that it was something that Jeff intended to throw out. I looked inside and found two pieces of toast, left over, I assumed, from one of his dinners.

"What should I do with this?" I asked. That's when the old memory emerged, and I laughed.

"Oh," I said, "I see you're still pulling no-toasters."

I laughed again, even more heartily, and at first Jeff didn't seem to get it but then I said,

"Remember the no-toasters" and he smiled, in that way. His old way.

"What so funny?" Dev asked.

"Oh," I answered. "Well, Dad always used to not like toast. I'd make some toast for me

and I'd say, 'Want some toast?' and Dad would say, 'No thanks' and I'd say 'Oh, you're pulling a no-toaster again' and we'd laugh." Jeff and I exchanged that kind of smile again.

Jeff nodded, in a smiley way, and we kissed again. His lips seemed soft and tender and magnetic and I didn't think about the teeth underneath them. How lately there was always food caught in the back. How a couple of visits before he had asked Devin to get out his toothbrush, and I had said, "I'm not brushing your teeth anymore." And he had said, "Just put the toothbrush in my mouth," and when I did he wriggled it around and seemed proud that he could take care of the lodged food by himself. And as I carried that toothbrush to the sink, ran it under the water, and beat it against the side of the sink, I closed my eyes. Like I sometimes did when I dealt with the suction tube.

I didn't think about all that. I just kissed him, then soon gave him another kiss good-bye 'til the next visit.

Marion Deutsche Cohen in the author of 17 books including the memoir *Dirty Details: The Days and Nights of a Well Spouse* (Temple University Press), *The Sitting-Down Hug* (The Liberal Press) and *Epsilon Country* (The Center for Thanatology Research). She is currently working on a sequel to *Dirty Details*. She is also a mathematician and author of *Crossing the Equal Sign* (Plain View Press), a new collection of poems about the experience of mathematics.

A Simple Gift
Courtney Taylor

What sort of gift do you present to a man who has spent 20 years in bed, immobilized from the neck down? Brendan, my boyfriend, was introducing me to his father, Wayne, who resided at Liberty Nursing Home, where multiple sclerosis had gradually disconnected his muscles from his mind. Told that his bed was next to a picture window, I settled on a sun catcher as my host's gift: a delicate spider web punched out of shiny brass, the spider's body a huge teardrop shaped crystal that reflected a dazzling rainbow of color in the light.

Like most nursing homes, Liberty had an oppressive odor of urine, fluorescent lighting, and patients, many elderly and confused. Wayne's roommate was a nearly deaf man whose Alzheimer's disease caused him, on occasion, to spontaneously call out the catch phrases of T.V. commercials. Sudden loud bursts of "Unclaimed Freight!" and "Crazy Eddie!" from behind the drawn curtain startled visitors in mid-conversation.

Brendan's father was alert and engaging. Buzz cut gray hair topped a remarkably unwrinkled and unblemished face that had been protected from years of sun damage and unnecessary facial expressions. For the most part, his head rested heavily on his chest, his neck muscles too weak to hold it up for long. MS had begun to furtively creep into his wide hazel eyes, causing them to quiver as they strained to focus. "Nice to make your acquaintance," Wayne said politely on that first visit. I struggled to understand his words, which rolled slowly around his tongue.

"I brought you a little something," I said.

"Thank you," he replied, eyeing the gold box wrapped in red ribbon placed on his tray table. Wayne's slender hands with their long, graceful fingers remained motionless on his belly.

"Here," Brendan intervened. "Let's open it up." Reaching across the bed, he tugged at the bow.

"Nice," Wayne crooned. "It's a spider. I like that."

"It's a sun catcher," I explained.

"I know," he drawled. "Put it up." Pressing the suction cup to the window, I looped the sun catcher's string over the hook. Prismatic color danced up the wall and across the ceiling. "Nice," Wayne repeated.

Wayne had spent his relatively happy childhood in a lush and hilly area of Pennsylvania, where small towns were joined by scenic expanses of Mennonite farms. A hitch in the army taught Wayne two important skills. One was drafting, which secured him a job with Atlas Battery immediately upon his return from the service. The other was picking up girls, and he soon fell hard for a pretty brunette on the Ferris wheel at a country fair.

Wayne and Dorene set up housekeeping and, from all accounts, lived blissfully for seven years. But shortly after the birth of Brendan, their only child, Wayne's journey into paralysis began. On Brendan's 12th birthday, Wayne tripped, shattering his hip and his shoulder. It was his last day at home. Weeks in the hospital and months in rehabilitation left little hope for his return.

Working full time and raising her son, Dorene could not adequately care for her increasingly debilitated husband. Now the man of the house, Brendan mowed the lawn and shoveled snow. Saturdays, instead of playing baseball, he wheelchair-raced his father down nursing home hallways. Eventually becoming too weak to spin the wheels, Wayne was transferred to Liberty. Brendan left for college and his mother divorced Wayne. Continuing her regular but less frequent visits with Wayne and handling his financial and practical affairs, she prodded her son to see his father more often after he returned from school.

When I moved in with Brendan, we had no need for a second T.V., so I offered mine to Wayne. He had an ancient and dust-infested clock radio that the nurses would tune to his favorite AM station that featured a conservative talk show host he liked and concerts by The Melody Aces, a local polka band. Wayne loved their cover of the Bobby Vinton hit "My Melody of Love." But his eyes lit up the day Brendan plugged in the television. One of the local stations carried reruns of sitcoms from the '60s and '70s: *The Andy Griffith Show*, *F Troop*, and *Little House on the Prairie* were his favorites. Episodes of *The Lawrence Welk Show* were broadcast on Saturday evenings. Gomer Pyle amused him, as did Lucy. Wayne welcomed them all like old friends.

> "In the end, pneumonia released Wayne from Liberty."

Of all the nurses, he liked Jennifer the best. With her knock-out smile and irreverent sense of humor, she brought Wayne breakfast from McDonald's before her shift. She smuggled in her husband's *Playboy* magazines and patiently turned the pages for Wayne to peruse the gorgeous unadorned bodies. He kept a photo of Jennifer and her two children on his bulletin board.

The *Sports Illustrated* swimsuit calendar hung beside the board. Each year we'd wrap it in festive holiday paper to present to him, then rip it off with anticipatory flair, flipping the months for him to preview. "Ni-ice," he'd remark. His quaking eyes studied each buxom babe while he noted their lovely differences and inquired about the exotic locales. One year he was particularly enamored of July. "Lemme see 'er again," he said. My husband turned back the months until he reached the glistening tan body in a wispy white bikini, sand glittering like diamonds around her as she stretched voluptuously on the beach. Long, wet, and disheveled brown curls clung seductively to one flushed cheek and foamy surf lapped at her bejeweled ankle. "Mmm-hmm," he crooned. "She's the best one. I like her." Then he'd let his chin drop to his chest, resting his strained eyes.

Sometimes Wayne's legs twitched uncontrollably. "Fix my feet," he'd say. Rolling back the covers at the bottom of the bed, one of us would refold the small square of sheepskin under his ankles and adjust his limp and atrophied legs. As I got to know Wayne better, I'd massage his feet gently for a few minutes, and he'd let his head fall back saying, "Ahhh, thas good."

Monthly haircuts and weekly baths administered by the staff kept Wayne fairly well groomed. But no one ever bothered to clean out the electric shaver kept in his bedside drawer. I took it upon myself to clean it thoroughly while Brendan read out loud *The Patriot*, Wayne's hometown weekly newspaper. The obituaries were of particular interest to Wayne. Brendan dutifully read the names and Wayne would say, "Nope ... nope ... don't know him," until Brendan got to one he recognized. "Yeayah," he'd say, cocking his head, "read that one." After finishing the article, Wayne added his own post-mortems: "She was in my class, not the prettiest girl." Or "One time he brought a chicken to school and put it under teacher's desk." Or, "He was at Atlas." They all opened up vivid, colorful, and, more often than not, hilarious tales.

While taking our leave, I'd hug Wayne. He'd respond with a kiss. Eventually, I added a kiss too, and began to plant it directly on his lips. "Thanks for the food," he'd say. "Thanks for the read. Thanks for the clean shaver."

"Okay, then," my husband would say awkwardly. "We'll see you soon." He rarely hugged his father.

"So long," was Wayne's standard sign-off. "Come again."

I only saw Wayne cry once. Brendan informed him that Dorene had died, succumbing to the chemotherapy that had successfully cured her brief bout with lymphoma, but had flooded her weakened heart. Wayne remained silent, his chin pushed far down on his chest, his eyes closed. After a long time, he lifted his head, his eyes misty. "That *is* sad news," he replied. Grief weighed down our lengthy silence until Wayne spoke up. He said, "I remember when she told me we were going to have a baby." He paused. He looked up at Brendan and said, "That was you."

In the end, pneumonia released Wayne from Liberty. Brendan stepped into the hallway of the hospital's I.C.U. to confer with the doctor. When he returned, he fiddled with the T.V. even though Wayne could not sit up or see it. Aunt Bea was consoling Opie after a bad day at school. I swabbed the inside of Wayne's mouth with water and Brendan wiped his father's burning brow with a cool washcloth.

"They want to insert a feeding tube," Brendan declared. Wayne turned his head to me, sheer terror in his eyes. "No oob, no oob" he gurgled insistently, struggling to lift his head off the pillow. "No tube," I echoed. "Okay, no tube," Brendan said and Wayne relaxed. A few minutes later Wayne garbled, "I onh oo iy, I onh oo iy." He repeated the syllables over and over, until it began to sound like "I want to die." Brendan and I exchanged nervous glances. Neither of us had the courage to repeat the words aloud. Exhausted by our refusal to comprehend, Wayne dropped his head and closed his eyes. Next to his bed, the monitors whirred. Curves began to straighten and numbers began to drop. Wayne's raspy and uneven breathing informed us of the battle being waged within. An hour elapsed, perhaps two.

Then, unexpectedly, Brendan lay down on the bed next to Wayne. One arm cradled his father's fevered head, the other reached across his belly. Nudging away the tubes, I lay down on the other side and closed my eyes. My ankle met Brendan's between his father's feet. By the time I opened my eyes, a golden October sun had silently stolen in through the window and crept up the bed, warmly blanketing the three of us.

Courtney Taylor is a freelance writer, handbag designer, and teacher. She holds a Bachelor of Arts degree in English and Art History from Connecticut College. She's currently resides in Medford, New Jersey with her beau and a cat called Abu.

Part V
The Gift of MS

Listing Port
Cynde Route

I was diagnosed with multiple sclerosis twelve years ago. I haven't had a relapse in several years, but not one hour—not one minute—passes when I'm unaware of it. I don't dwell on it, but it's with me in the back of my mind all the time: *I have a disease. I have multiple sclerosis.* I don't want MS, but I can't deny that while it has taken some things away from me that I'll probably never get back, coping with MS has given me unimaginable gifts, gifts that I could not have attained without the sacrifice.

Here's one of the things I've sacrificed: I can't run. I ran infrequently in the old days, never more than a couple of times a week for two or three-month stretches, and never further than five miles. I didn't like it much, so I don't think I would have evolved into a runner by now, even if I could run. But I would like to be able to run a little bit, to my car from the grocery store in a sudden rain, for example. But I can't. I can think about it, though, and I do. You should see me run in my dreams! I'm one of those people who remembers her dreams nearly every day. For the most part, they feature me in an endless variety of ridiculous situations that seem perfectly normal in the dream. But my running dreams are always the same: I am trying to catch someone, like a long-lost friend who's disappeared in a crowd. I walk faster and faster as I try to catch up to the person until, suddenly, I'm running. It turns out that I *can* run. Fast. In the dream, I always make a mental note to tell Michael, my husband, that I can run, as soon as I catch the person I'm after. Then I wake up.

I guess thinking about running is like thinking about wiggling my ears: I can think about it all day long, but my ears won't wiggle. And my legs won't run. Mark Twain said that a man who doesn't read good books has no advantage over a man who can't read them, and I guess the same is true for a woman who can't run. Plenty of people don't ever run, anyway. (Oh, I'd like to take the stairs two at a time once in a while, too. And I *would* jump rope, if I could.)

Another thing MS has taken away from me is my balance. I'm certain that to most people I look steady enough. To my family and friends, I might look a little unbalanced sometimes. But to me, I feel on the verge of falling, well, most of the time. I have to think about each step when I walk across a room. If there is something that I can simply touch—a chair back, a countertop—then I'm okay. I dread having to stand up and cross an open space, but sometimes it can't be avoided. I try to prepare myself first by stretching my legs and getting the kinks out of my ankles. Then, focused on my goal, I just do it.

> "You should see me run in my dreams!"

I like to grocery shop because of the cart; I don't feel even a little shaky as long as I have a cart to hold on to. My chivalrous sons and husband feel about as foolish walking beside me in the store while I push the cart as they would if I were carrying a fifty-pound bag of Purina while they strolled along unencumbered. But they know that it helps me to have the cart, so they don't insist on taking it from me.

I can't walk a straight line to save my life. I describe myself as listing port, because I always seem to veer off to the left. If I were ever stopped by the police and asked to walk a line, they'd take one look at my unsteady gait and assume I was drunk. I'll go pretty far out of my way to avoid even a little bit of ice or snow or mud, because stepping in it might break my self-imposed rhythm.

My balance issue, as I refer to it, bothers me more than any other symptom of MS because it has the potential to make me appear frail, which I'm not. I try to project myself to the world as the strong, capable woman that I am inside, but one or two faltering steps could destroy that picture. I don't want anyone to feel sorry for me; pity from other people implies a fragility in me that I don't feel. What bothers me about my balance isn't my potential for falling—I can accept that—it's what witnessing a fall, or even a stagger, would induce in other people. One snowy winter night, my husband Michael and I went to see my middle son's chorus concert. After the show, Michael went to get the car, and my son and I decided to walk out to it rather than wait. As we made our way through the crowd of teens and parents streaming from the building, Peter stepped off the curb and turned to offer his arm.

"Peter, what a sweet thing for you to do!" I exclaimed as I took hold of him. He shot back, "Mom, do you have any idea how embarrassing it would be for me if you fell *right here*?" Now that's the attitude I like. Peter wasn't helping me because he thought I was weak; he was just trying to avoid his own embarrassment, the way any teenager would.

That brings me to the gifts MS has given me. I guess everybody loves their children and thinks they're the best kids ever, but mine really are. My twelve year-old daughter was only four months old when I was diagnosed, and my seventeen and eighteen year-old sons were just little boys. They've grown up knowing that they always have to consider me, unlike most kids, who can think first of themselves. I believe that because of this, my children take other people into consideration, too. They're thoughtful and attentive to their friends, their teachers, even the guy who drives their school bus. No one has to carry anything when they're around. They model their behavior after their father, who always treats me with compassion and respect, but never pity.

We have always enjoyed wilderness canoeing, and though there are portages—hikes from one lake to the next where the canoes and all the gear have to be carted—I never carry anything. When planning a canoe trip, my family's main concern is not whether or not they can transport the canoes and our belongings over a long portage, but whether I can walk that far. In camp, I don't have to do anything. Along with Michael, the kids cook, clean, set up the tents, and pack everything up again when it's time to leave. Imagine canoeing and camping while being treated as if you're in a luxury hotel. That's what MS has given me.

Finally, having MS has given me my health. If it sounds like a contradiction to say a disease has given me my health, consider that coping with MS has caused me not only to monitor my physical status continually, but to assess my own efforts toward improving it. Since my diagnosis, I have eaten a primarily vegan diet—no dairy, no meat, no hydrogenated fat—because I learned about the connections between saturated fat and MS early on. I take a handful of carefully selected vitamins every day. I get plenty of sleep each night. I lift weights at my local gym every other day. I am strong and fit and I'm thinner than I was in high school. My bad cholesterol is low and my good cholesterol is high. I'm never sick; if not for the fact that I have MS, I'd be in perfect health!

I don't leave anything up to chance where my health is concerned. Just like my children automatically do the right thing, I automatically do the healthy thing. I'm a 44 year-old woman and I'm in the best shape of my life. I guess it's wrong to say that MS has given me my health. Rather, I should say that because of MS, I've taken it. If I were never diagnosed with it, would I be an overweight, out of shape woman with bratty kids and low self-esteem?

I don't know, but I am the person that I am because of what life has given me to work with, and among other things, it's given me multiple sclerosis.

_____

As she puts it, Cynde Route is an utterly non-technical composition instructor at a technical college. She bakes pies, makes soup, reads lots of books, and plants flowers. She has homeschooled her children, taught Lamaze, and given birth at home. She moves at a slow pace while the world rushes around her.

My MS Rollercoaster
Alba Barton

Rollercoaster. That's the word that describes my relationship with multiple sclerosis. I have "up" days when I'm feeling normal, on top of the world, invincible, happy and forget that I even have it. I also have "steady" days when everything is going fine and my list of complaints is very small. I may have a little bump or two, but I deal with it and move on. And of course, I have "down" days when I'm feeling not only emotionally but physically drained. I rant and rave. My temper is shorter than usual and my depression can get pretty deep. It's days like those that can be pretty frightening. Those are the days when I allow MS to get the best of me. But that doesn't happen very often, nor does it last very long.

I haven't told many people about my disease, mostly because I can't bear to watch their expressions change, first to shock and then pity. I would say that "I don't look like I have MS," but what does a person with MS look like? Is it a person in a wheelchair? Using a cane? Bedridden? No. A person with MS looks like your neighbor, your postal carrier, your child's teacher, or a marathon runner. It can be any one of the people you see every day. Not everyone who has MS has visible signs of disability or even the same symptoms as anyone else. Some look perfectly healthy on the outside. I am one of those people. I'll never forget the comment my neurologist made when he came into the exam room the first day we met. He looked at me after looking at my MRI's and said, "Wow! You look great for someone who has over 60 lesions on her brain." I chuckle whenever I remember that day.

One thing is for certain, though. MS didn't know what it was in for when it invaded my body. I don't have time for it. I have three teenagers that keep me busy. I have to be alert, quick-witted and always two steps ahead of them. I have a husband who is active in sports and fitness, which in turn keeps me fit and on my toes. I also work out at the gym six days a week. I have laundry to wash, dinner to cook, errands to run and a house that seems to need cleaning all the time. In addition, I have to have time for emergencies and things that just pop up. My days are completely booked. I won't let MS interfere with my life. I can't afford it.

> "A person with MS looks like your neighbor, your postal carrier, your child's teacher, or a marathon runner."

Fortunately for me, my MS has not been overly demanding of my time. It has not yet become selfish to the point of rendering me disabled. Sure, I think about my MS progressing, but that doesn't stop me from living my life. When I feel discouraged and frightened, I become angry. Angry at the disease and the havoc it wreaks on my mind, body and spirit. It not only affects me but also my family. It's then that I become focused and determined to fight it every step of the way.

My family keeps me grounded. My husband is my biggest supporter and champion. Sometimes, his faith in me surpasses my own. I can trust that he will never let me give up, no matter how dire things may get. My family tells me that I am brave. My friends say that I'm a driving force. It's difficult for me to see what they see. I'm just living my life and taking it all in stride. MS hasn't stopped me yet. Trust me when I say that I refuse to go down without a fight. Things may get ugly, but I plan to give it a run for its money.

Alba Barton was diagnosed with multiple sclerosis in 2001. She resides in Waxham, North Carolina with Marc, her husband of 17 years. She has three children, Ashley, Aaron and Jesslyn.

Tough Year
Caryl Yvonne Hunter

It had already been a tough year. It had been month after month of choices made for me. A constant hemorrhaging that could only be stopped by a hysterectomy and the end of any possibility of having a child—and with it the reminder of the child I'd lost years earlier. Then the change of heart from my then-husband, who decided he no longer wanted to be married. And now this.

The darkness in my left eye was too much to bear. My vision was getting increasingly blurry. I tried to tell myself it was an allergic reaction or stress. Eventually everything looked like an old black and white negative, then black. Nothing. The pain that went with it was so strong that I could barely turn my head. I convinced myself it was some sort of extreme migraine. It was a disorienting and violent pounding. The pain made it hard to walk without aggravating my eye and I was dizzy and clumsy. I convinced my husband to take me to the emergency room.

Once there, I waited for hours, my husband impatiently looking at his watch every few minutes and rolling his eyes when mine teared up with pain. When I finally saw a doctor hours later, I was told, "I want you to see an ophthalmologist who specializes in things like this." Things like this? Like what?

"I don't think this is a migraine," The doctor continued. "There is a condition that happens to young women, usually in the northern states. It's called optic neuritis. It's an inflammation of the optic nerve behind your eye. I want you to get over to see this guy right away. He's the best in this field."

The ophthalmologist commented that the ER doctor had been correct in his assessment and I was extremely lucky he had caught it. He recommended I see a neurologist right away, adding that I shouldn't worry. Sure, Doc. When I saw a nurse to schedule the appointment, she was very helpful:

"We'll get you in to see a neurologist at Methodist. Do you have MS then?"

"What?" I was shocked. "No, just optic neuritis."

It seemed like forever until I got to the neurologist, although it was only a couple of days. But time passes slowly when you're hurting, afraid and alone. My husband, already out of the marriage emotionally, virtually disappeared. He would not drive me to the doctor, so my driving was very slow, bumping off curbs and taking side roads. My left eye completely blind, I crept into the right lane and stayed there.

The neurology appointment was anything but routine, and an MRI was ordered as well as daily visits to the hospital for intravenous Prednisone treatments. Too embarrassed by my husband's behavior to tell anyone or ask a friend, I endured it all on my own. My mouth tasted like metal and the high levels of Prednisone made me puffy and irritable. I was told to rest as much as possible, but the pain was too intense.

My appointment to get the MRI results was on a bright, sunny day. With my vision so different in each eye, the bright sun made driving even more arduous. My right eye was also starting to feel the strain from doing all the work. After a long, scary drive, I arrived at the doctor's office to see my MRI films, which were already hanging in his office with a light behind them. There were large white patches all over the film. "These are scans of your brain," she said. "I'm sorry, but the white patches show that you do have multiple sclerosis." She explained the myelin sheaths. She explained the treatment. She said she wanted to see me again. But it was all a blur. I cried all the way home.

> "My trials have taught me compassion toward other people I wouldn't trade for anything now."

What I needed more than anything was the husband I had married many years earlier to greet me on my return. But when I walked in to be greeted by my husband's cruel indifference, I knew right then that the husband I'd married no longer existed, and the marriage was over. I made a long distance call to my parents later that evening to get the support I so needed. "I can't believe it. It has been such a horrible year. I can't take this on top of everything else."

"I know, honey." My mom said quietly. "We are so sorry."

The good news was that my eye did eventually respond to treatment. After a couple of months, my eyesight slowly returned. My right eye went dark soon after, but that too responded to medication. The right eye was not as severe or as painful, and my left eye still remains the more vulnerable one.

I still have remittent multiple sclerosis and have had other episodes of optic neuritis. And I still have eye pain, headaches, extreme fatigue, and feel pins and needles in my legs and feet. I'm still unsteady at times and have difficulty in severe heat. But I'm fortunate that I respond well to medication. And I'm most fortunate that I'm now living a healthy and happy life.

Once my eyes were truly opened, I saw many things more clearly than I ever had. I got out of the miserable relationship I hadn't been happy in for years. After several years on my own, I've done more than I ever would have staying married. I graduated from college with honors with only one eye "working." I've traveled all over the world. And I now work in a social services field, fortunate to help others with their own health problems that I would not have understood fully until I went through my own. My trials have taught me compassion toward other people I wouldn't trade for anything now. Dealing with the challenges of MS has helped me become a stronger, more independent woman. I know now that it is only through my darkest journey that I've truly learned to appreciate the light.

Caryl Yvonne Hunter is a freelance writer and photographer living in Minneapolis, Minnesota. She also works in the social services field in outreach programs throughout the Twin Cities area.

Balancing on Pins and Needles
Sonia Rice

These days, I look at my life as "before diagnosis" and "after diagnosis." I'm 59 years old, in my fourth year after diagnosis. I consider myself extremely lucky that I was able to live a "normal" life up to age 55. Let's call it "relatively normal" because I had decades of unresolved and what seemed to be ridiculous medical symptoms before I was diagnosed. No doctor I saw about them mentioned MS as a possibility, and since I knew nothing about the disease, I certainly never thought about it. I think about it all the time now, except that I don't really "think" about it. It's more like a constant companion: it's with me all day, every day.

Before my diagnosis, my symptoms were innocuous enough, stuff that would come and go. Some episodes lasted longer and caused more disability than others. I would make my way to chiropractors and doctors who spoke to me about degenerative disc disease, arthritis, other aging conditions and nothing much to worry my pretty little head about. So I went about my life, running my own company, raising two daughters. I had two marriages, two divorces, extended family, and wonderful friends. I went on vacations, I volunteered my time to various organizations, and I enjoyed my hobbies. I even beat malignant melanoma when I was 36 and pregnant. It was a "normal" life.

But I realize now that I should have known something was terribly wrong that summer four years ago. I felt a drastic change in my energy level. Many afternoons, I would close the door to my office and lie on the floor to nap. While before I could easily walk miles along the Atlantic City boardwalk and play for hours in the ocean, I could barely walk the short distance to the beach without feeling exhausted. I would ask myself, *am I working too hard?* I rationalized it away by chalking it all up to stress.

The rationalizing ended one Sunday morning when I woke with severe pain in my right shoulder. Over the next few days I began to lose feeling above and below my elbow and in my hand. I self-diagnosed: *must be that trick neck of mine going out again.* I went to the chiropractor. After three weeks of nearly daily treatments, I could barely move my right hand and when I did, sharp "electric" shocks and severe pain would run up my hand and arm into my shoulder. Since using the computer was an integral part of my work, the pain was constant and excruciating. I could handle some pain, but this made me cry.

Over the next few months I saw my primary care physician, had an MRI, got referred to a neurologist, had more tests, got another MRI, and then, at last, I got a second opinion that finally yielded a diagnosis: *multiple sclerosis.* It was the end of my life as I knew it.

My first reaction was to take my diagnosis in my typical "Type A" stride: this disease wasn't going to run *me.* But even though I was determined not to let this disease take over, my life did change drastically. Over the next months, food became uninteresting to me, which was unnerving, since I'm one of those "live to eat" people and cooking has always been a passion. My 5'9", size 12 body soon shrank to a size 4. You would assume I would be happy about my new body, but I could see how frightened my children, family, and close friends were at my unhealthy appearance. Most days I didn't have the energy to get out of bed. I survived on cranberry juice and an occasionally nibble on toasted cheese sandwiches.

Eventually I made a goal of getting out of bed and doing one thing each day, even if it meant showering at 5 P.M. But in addition to the MS (or because of it), I was also depressed and angry about having no control over what was happening to me. I was seeing a therapist, but it was extraordinarily difficult facing a future fraught with such limitations.

My condition influenced me to make decisions that were both good and not so good. Ending my 35-year career was a good one because I could no longer be effective at my job. It required too much concentration, and the fatigue kept me from being reliable. I fell down the stairs of my townhouse three times and decided to sell it and move to a condominium. At the time, it seemed to be the right decision, but my personality isn't suited to condo living and I soon knew that this was not going to be a permanent situation. My townhouse was lovely and maybe I could have made modifications so that I could be safe in that environment.

I also learned how expensive a disease like MS can be. Many of us aren't able to work, so paying for our wonderful disease-modifying drugs can be impossible. You may have disability insurance through your employer or private disability insurance. If you've paid into Social Security your entire career, you may be entitled to benefits that cover these expenses. Try not to get frustrated or frightened. Take it one step at a time and don't give up.

In the four years since my diagnosis, I've learned to look at life quite differently. Stress is stress, so I avoid it whenever I can. I'm always balancing my energy with the commitments I've made. If an activity gets added, something else usually has to be deleted. I try not to over-commit, but I do my best to keep the commitments that I do make, since keeping our circle of friends is very important. Because many MS symptoms are invisible, there have been times when our friends haven't understood what's happening to me. MS doesn't necessarily make you look "sick", and sometimes people naturally assume that my MS-induced fatigue is just like the fatigue they feel after a long day. Dealing with these misperceptions takes some getting used to, but I've found that my true friends are just that, and they'll always be there.

Complementary healthcare makes me feel better. Weekly acupuncture helps with pain and energy. Physical therapy tones my muscles. A class called Moving with Ease helped me to understand that sometimes we just need to put our brains in gear to move. This helps most when the fatigue gets overwhelming. My ability to concentrate isn't anywhere close to what it was, my neurogenic bladder becomes unmanageable when I'm overtired. I often have headaches, unexplained pain, constant pins and needles in my arms and legs, strange twitches, and more. The latest symptom is that my right foot starts to drag after I've walked for five to ten minutes. But even with these difficulties, and living with the knowledge that my condition could change at any time, I feel grateful—grateful for my family, my friends old and new, my partner Richard, the MS Society in Delaware that is caring, supportive, accessible, and helps so many of us in so many ways. I'm most grateful for my own resilience and my ability to love my life.

> "I've found that my true friends are just that, and they'll always be there."

While MS is a horrible disease, having it presents an opportunity to assess where you are in your life. It can help you to get to know your real strengths, to be your true self, and to make conscious choices about how you spend your days.

Before her diagnosis, Sonia Rice was President of The Breakthrough Communications Group, an award winning marketing and communications company located in Wilmington, Delaware. She is the proud mother of Jill and Paula and the unmeddling mother-in-law of Peter.

The Gift of MS

Bonni Barcus

Being diagnosed with multiple sclerosis has unlocked my life and given me more happiness than I ever thought possible for a girl raised on a dirt farm in Iowa by Depression-era grandparents. I have come to believe that my MS is a gift, and without it, my life would not be as full and rich as it is today.

When I was diagnosed after experiencing numbness, tingling, and weakness down my whole left side, I had the expected reaction of someone who has just found out that an incurable disease is in her life: I was devastated. Or was I? I didn't feel mentally different. I was still me, only with tingles. I could still do anything I used to do, only with some irritating numbness in my limbs and the "ants" crawling on my skin and scalp. It could be worse, and would be in time, but for now, this wasn't so bad.

If hard life on the farm taught me anything, it was that you made hay while the sun shone, and when it was cloudy, you could always bake bread. After a week or so of mulling the possible outcomes of having MS and envisioning worst-case scenarios of the next 30 years or so, I did what any "Type A" personality would do: I took inventory. What could I do now that I might not be able to do in the future? What would I regret not trying? I realized very quickly that there were no guarantees of a sunny tomorrow, and it was haying time *today*.

I made a list of things I'd always wanted to try. I had always loved stained glass. I took a class once a week through the community college and learned to make some wonderful things. I camped, hiked, and bought my first house, an old Victorian needing a lot of TLC—the first of six homes I would tackle. I found that knocking out a wall or ripping up a floor gave me an outlet for the frustration that crept in on a regular basis. Sometimes it just felt good to tear something up and rebuild it. The therapy of taking a worn out house and breathing new life into it also renewed my spirits and did good things for the neighborhood.

One day a friend asked me to go downhill skiing. *Skiing?* I had never even given it a thought, and it wasn't on my list! But with my new attitude, I said "Why not? What's the worst that can happen?" With MS, I feel more active when I'm cooler, and the thought of getting outdoors was very appealing. We went skiing on a Saturday, and I somehow managed to stop and turn within a couple of hours, and we headed to the top of the mountain to take a beginner trail down. I was hooked from the very first minute. My hair froze to my coat in the icy rain that started to fall by noon, and I was glazed in ice. It took us two hours to reach the lodge at the bottom, and when we arrived, the weather was lousy enough to close the ski resort. I walked into the lodge with ice cracking off my coat and hair feeling elated! I could not stop smiling.

What freedom! I could slide and glide, the views were breathtaking, the fresh air was rejuvenating and with enough practice, I found I could ski better than I walked at times, and this empowered me. Instead of being cooped up in a house when it snowed, I got in the car and drove to the ski hill. Being a single mom, I took my ten-year-old daughter with me and we learned together.

Over the next few years, my skills were improving even as my balance was going in the opposite direction. This would not do! I didn't want to give up my new favorite winter activity so soon. I wasn't ready to stay in and bake bread just yet, but the clouds were rolling in. So I went online to get more information on skiing and found Epicski.com, and this was the start of yet another new life for me. I met my husband, a ski patroller, on this website and we have been happily married now for four years. We have found that life in our 50s is more full than life at 20, with so many mountains and so little time to ski them.

Through Epicski, I have met others who ski and I've taken lessons with other enthusiastic members of the ski community. They boost my spirits and listen to me whine, and encourage me when I'm down. I'm skiing a little slower these days, but I get a boost when I see people in their 80s slowly winding their way down the mountain with smiles on their faces. Some days it's better to do that jigsaw puzzle instead of go out and ski, but when the days are good, I go out and play. I know I'll be skiing as long as I can stay on my feet. I am truly thankful that MS entered my world and got me to stop taking life for granted.

> "I am truly thankful that MS entered my world and got me to stop taking life for granted."

Warren Miller, a ski filmmaker, once said, "If you don't do it this year, you'll be one year older when you do." He's absolutely right. There's no time like the present to learn new skills and to have some fun. You can bake bread any day, but it's haying time today.

Bonni Barcus is 52, an avid skier, gardener and home remodeler. She's had MS for 15 years. She and her husband live in Massachusetts, but are considering moving to ski country for retirement.

My Part-Time Job

Gayle Franck

Competent. Detached. Maybe a little curious. This was my attitude when, as a young registered nurse, I first met patients with
multiple sclerosis. There was the middle-aged homebound man
whose arm muscle spasms caused him to cry out in pain; I com-
plied with his request to massage this distress, buried deeply in his
bicep. There was the elderly paraplegic woman's gastric tube feeding while she lay in the long-term care facility, the picture of health
in every way but for the tube. Another young man, whose disease
progressed especially rapidly, was convinced that diet and nutrition were the only keys to a cure.

I listened to their frustrations and found what solutions I could for
vague complaints. I adjusted therapies, brainstormed with physicians, and helped fine-tune medication orders to best meet physical, emotional or financial needs.

For a decade, my nursing days were filled with the challenges of
part-time work with four area agencies while I raised our four children. I felt privileged to experience a variety of nursing and administrative perspectives. From the premature infant to the
twenty-something woman with melanoma to the elderly dialysis
recipient, my learning and caring opportunities seemed limitless.
However, my own diagnosis of MS gave me a new part-time job:

taking care of myself. Administrative excellence, determination and persistence are important for success in this responsibility as well.

One winter evening, my husband and I were sprinting through the rain to the theater. Suddenly a strange electric feeling tightened the muscles of my left thigh, and I limped into the lobby. I forgot about the incident until later that winter, when I noticed a return of the sensation. I ignored this, too, but within a few weeks I was unable to walk more than a block without the leg seizing up. Then, the "stocking" numbness occurred: both legs, while functional, were numb from the knees down.

I consulted a physician. In the examining room, the doctor and a medical student acknowledged that it seemed the vibratory sense of the nerves in my legs was that of a seventy-year-old. I was forty-two. Imagine my confusion, when moments later, I overheard the two of them discussing the possibility of referring me to a psychiatrist. Dumbfounded, I waited on the other side of the closed door while they whispered.

My mind raced back to psychiatric nursing classes. I remembered the admonition to rule out some symptoms as psychosomatic, especially if they occur bilaterally and sporadically. This concept was softened by the condescending tone of the nursing text: "Of course, the symptom is real to the patient, so it must be addressed with empathy...."

Was I delusional? No. After several MRIs, a neurologist diagnosed MS. A series of consults with many specialists, and therapies and hospitalizations resulted in some symptoms retreating over the years. Or, was I in temporary remission? No one could tell. A few new symptoms emerged. Was the MS getting worse? Again, there were no easy answers. Characteristically, one constant with this autoimmune disease was fatigue.

For me, fatigue has been the one unchanging symptom. It never seems to vary much in onset or duration between many daily instances: every 1½ to 4 hours, with approximately 20–60 minutes of rest for recovery (reclining). However, other symptoms are as varied as the tissues enervated by damaged myelin-encased nerves. Wherever the insulating myelin sheath is "sclerosed" (damaged or missing), impulses can be distorted or weakened–hence, the wide variety of symptoms.

Today, as I have for the 17 years since my diagnosis, I carve out time for this new part-time work. Sometimes, the relentless routines of self-care threaten my resolve. Sometimes, I even reconsider whether to show up for "work." *I'll skip it just once, I think. I'm tired of that boring stuff; I've called my own holiday; I've decided to take a day off.* Several hours later, the familiar stiffness starts climbing up my limbs and my back. *Uh oh. I will pay for this indiscretion.* So the next morning I dutifully report to my job. I know I can't risk two days off. In my living room, I begin the routine taught to me by my physical therapist. Stretch the legs, lower back, this way and that. Hold each stretch for thirty seconds (I usually don't). Sit ups, first straight and then diagonally. Twenty-one times. As the clock above the piano marks thirty minutes, I have almost completed the stretching exercises. I am feeling more flexible, but now I have to do the strength training.

> "Whatever is required to keep going, I will attempt to find the best solution and adapt to a constantly changing physical environment."

I grab the three-pound weighted dumbbells and start the arm lifts. I think, *How can I make the aerobic exercise interesting today?* Lacking an indoor pool, I decide to walk the neighborhood in an unfamiliar direction. I will try to include some gentle hill climbing. If the weather is bad, I suppose I could do the stairs again, or the exercise bike in the basement.

When I add up the time spent in stretching, aerobic and strength-building exercises with intermittent rest periods, it seems to average about four hours a day. While that is a chunk of anybody's time, it actually means I can buy more time for myself. Four hours a day pays me with a normal life for the remaining hours. There are other intangible benefits. People assume I have stamina, so that's very cool. When I attend continuing education events, or university classes, or perform my music, other people don't have to know that I will bookend my activity with rest. "You look great!" they will say, and I don't have to respond, "I should, I just bounced out of bed." Of course, if I am so brazen as to believe this charade and keep on going, a curious thing will happen. As I socialize or concentrate, my eyes will reveal the fatigue that is creeping up on me. If the minutes stretch on with my "normal behavior," other MS symptoms will gently remind me that they are waiting in the wings, should I choose to resist resting. When I ignore this and push them aside, MS will pull rank, and I am reminded that to flaunt its authority is foolishness. Cloudy vision, increasing arm numbness, and even moodiness will slowly force the issue of "break time."

MS hasn't been such a bad boss. The tedium gets frustrating, but there are benefits. Even resting has its advantages. Never have I been so good at prioritizing time and energy. Schedules are more predictable, and thus more efficient. Before MS, I jumbled so many things together into my days that there seemed to be little productivity. Now I have time to think, to meditate, to write. I have time to read and time to study.

Missing myelin may cause temporary setbacks and minor short circuits of sensation and endurance, but this has forced me to focus on my strengths. I can contribute RN knowledge and insight in a variety of settings. Even while bedridden for a time, I was able to homeschool our children. The local library provided help with their homebound programs, and today computers bring the world to me in infinite ways. When I worked for those nursing agencies, I never balked at embracing new technologies or medication delivery procedures. I did not complain about changing administrative or managerial requirements as I switched from agency to agency, even within a week's time. Why succumb to a stale or rigid mindset now, while administering my own health needs? Whatever is required to keep going, I will attempt to find the best solution and adapt to a constantly changing physical environment.

While optic neuritis necessitates tinted eyeglasses at times, at least I can look fashionable during classes. Using a scooter gives me extra hours of stamina to view museum exhibits or to explore a scenic outdoor trail. Fatigue's price may be no more than settling into a rocker to enjoy an infant's searching gaze. Stiff limbs simply force me to get up and engage in life. When out walking and a neighbor comments on my commitment to exercise, I feel like an athlete. Even a dash of self pity serves its purpose, encouraging empathy with fellow sufferers.

However, there will be no retirement now; taking care of myself is a day-to-day investment in my future. My commitment will pay off in multiple ways, as I look forward to continued learning and sharing proactive perspectives in healthcare. Whether in the university, community or family setting, wellness is always a priority. For me—personally—it will always be my part-time job.

Gayle Franck lives in Batavia, Illinois, where she and her husband raised four children. After retiring from nursing, she earned her Bachelor's degree and is currently working on her Master's degree. She is a music volunteer at church and in healthcare settings. Every week, she and her husband Joe are privileged to babysit their eight grandchildren, so life is never boring and she has to keep moving!

Finding My Voice

Roxanne D. Marion

I called it my "cute walk."

I had invented it so as to not worry my students. The walk consisted of slowly striding down the hall, close to the wall, keeping my hand near it to make sure I would catch myself if I lost my balance.

Then there was the constant tingling in my arms and legs, usually either on one side or the other. I had a solution for this one as well, especially when I had to drive. I would set the cruise control and let whichever side needed it at the time, rest. If my arm seemed too heavy, I would let it rest on my leg and keep the other tingling arm on the bottom of the steering wheel. The only "onset" of the MS I could not hide was the constant tripping, which I later found out was called foot drop. This is when your foot seems too heavy to pick up. You trip. A lot.

The first time I went to physical therapy, the therapist sat down with me and asked many questions about what my work days consisted of. When I told her that Saturdays were my cleaning days, she told me that I could no longer have one cleaning day. She suggested that I would now have to rearrange my long-held cleaning routine. She said I would not be able to accomplish multiple larger tasks, but instead I would have to mix one large and one small task, such as dusting with laundry or cleaning the bathroom with folding clothes. This was to help lower the stress on my body, which would then help me defer fatigue.

In that moment, I felt like I was losing control. Looking back, now, though, I see that my diagnosis of MS, ironically, gave me strength. Its hard necessities allowed me to find that voice within that said, "Yes I can," when everyone else was reminding me of what I could not do anymore. I still hear that voice inside me that says, "You can do it, you just have to try." Yes, I listen to my doctors, but I also listen to my own voice because I know "me" better than anyone can. If I had given up on in this journey with multiple sclerosis, the disease would have had me. Now I control it, and am happy to say what many MS patients say:

> "I may have MS, but MS does not have me!"

"I may have MS, but MS does not have me!"

Roxanne Marion, is a teacher raised in Indiana and now residing in Augusta, Georgia.

Resources

Listed below you will find information on some of the foremost organizations focused on providing information, treatment and care for persons meeting the challenges of livng with multiple sclerosis and their families and friends.

Information

National Multiple Sclerosis Society
National Capital Chapter
1800 M Street, N.W.
Suite 750 South
Washington, D.C. 20036
Telephone: (202) 296-5363
To find the chapter closest to you, dial 800-344-4867 (800 FIGHT MS) and your call will be regionally routed
www.nationalmssociety.org

The National MS Society is a collective of passionate individuals who want to do something about MS now—to move together toward a world free of multiple sclerosis. MS stops people from moving. NMSS exists to make sure it doesn't.

NMSS helps each person address the challenges of living with MS through its 50-state network of chapters. The Society helps people affected by MS by funding cutting-edge research, driving change through advocacy, facilitating professional education, and providing programs and services that help people with MS and their families move their lives forward.

National Institute of Neurological Disorders and Stroke
NIH Neurological Institute
P.O. Box 5801
Bethesda, MD 20824
Telephone: (800) 352-9424 or (301) 496-5751
www.ninds.nih.gov

The mission of NINDS is to reduce the burden of neurological disease—a burden borne by every age group, by every segment of society, by people all over the world. To support this mission, NINDS conducts, fosters, coordinates, and guides research on the causes, prevention, diagnosis, and treatment of neurological disorders and stroke, and supports basic research in related scientific areas, provides grants-in-aid to public and private institutions and individuals in fields related to its areas of interest, including research project, program project, and research center grants, conducts research in its own laboratories, branches, and clinics, and collects and disseminates research information related to neurological disorders.

The Mayo Clinic.com
www.mayoclinic.com/

Mayo Clinic is the first and largest integrated, not-for-profit group practice in the world. Doctors from every medical specialty work together to care for patients, joined by common systems and a philosophy of "the needs of the patient come first." More than 3,300 physicians, scientists and researchers and 46,000 allied health staff work at Mayo Clinic, which has sites in Rochester, Minnesota, Jacksonville, Florida, and Scottsdale/Phoenix, Arizona Collectively, the three locations treat more than half a million people each year. The Mayo Clinic.com provides an in-depth explanation of MS, its causes, treatment and outlook for the future.

Multiple Sclerosis Foundation
6350 North Andrews Avenue
Fort Lauderdale, Florida 33309-2130
Telephone: (800) 225-6495
www.msfacts.org

A predominantly service-based, non-profit organization, The Multiple Sclerosis Foundation provides a comprehensive approach to helping people with MS maintain both their health and well-being. We offer programming and support to keep them self-sufficient and their homes safe, while our educational programs heighten public awareness and promote understanding about the illness.

Multiple Sclerosis International Federation
3rd Floor Skyline House
200 Union Street
London
SE1 0LX
Telephone: +44 (0) 20 7620 1911
www.msif.org

The Multiple Sclerosis International Federation (MSIF) was established in 1967 as an international body linking the activities of national MS societies around the world. Its mission is to lead the global MS movement to improve the quality of life of people affected by MS and to support better understanding and treatment of MS by facilitating international cooperation between MS societies, the international research community and other stakeholders. It works to achieve this through international research, the development of new and existing societies, the exchange of information and advocacy.

Multiple Sclerosis Association of America
706 Haddonfield Road
Cherry Hill, NJ 08002
(800) 532-7667
www.msassociation.org

The Multiple Sclerosis Association of America (MSAA) is a national nonprofit organization dedicated to enriching the quality of life for everyone affected by multiple sclerosis. MSAA provides ongoing support and direct services to these individuals with MS and the people close to them. MSAA also serves to promote greater understanding of the needs and challenges of those who face physical obstacles.

In addition to a variety of programs and services—such as consultations, support groups, equipment distribution, MRI diagnostic funding, and public awareness campaigns—MSAA also provides valuable information through its quarterly magazine and other literature.

The American Autoimmune Related Diseases Association
National Office:
22100 Gratiot Ave.
East Detroit, MI 48021
Telephone: (586)776.3900
www.aarda.org

The American Autoimmune Related Diseases Association is dedicated to the eradication of autoimmune diseases and the alleviation of suffering and the socioeconomic impact of autoimmunity through fostering and facilitating collaboration in the areas of education, public awareness, research, and patient services in an effective, ethical and efficient manner.

National Association for Continence
P.O. Box 8310
Spartanburg, SC 29305-8310
(800) BLADDER
(864) 579-7900
www.nafc.org

NAFC is the largest and most prolific consumer education and advocacy organization dedicated to bladder and bowel health. Its website provides information on what you should know, when you should seek help, and what to ask your physician.

USA.gov
www.usa.gov

A comprehensive, A to Z listing of virtually every government agency providing information on multiple sclerosis, government research, benefits programs, financial aid, veteran's affairs information, and much more.

Treatment

Cleveland Clinic Mellon Center for
Multiple Sclerosis Treatment and Research
9500 Euclid Avenue
Cleveland, Ohio 44195
Telephone: (800)223.2273
www.clevelandclinicmeded.com

As part of the Cleveland Clinic's Neurological Institute, the Mellen Center for Multiple Sclerosis offers state-of-the-art resources to provide the most advanced specialized care, supported by an extensive program of research and education. The Mellen Center is the largest and most comprehensive program for MS care and research worldwide, managing more than 20,000 patient visits every year. Basic and clinical research conducted at the Cleveland Clinic sheds new light on MS every year.

The center's mission is to provide patients and their families compassionate, comprehensive, innovative and technologically advanced care of the highest quality, to conduct clinical and basic research of national and international distinction, and to educate clinicians, academicians, investigators and allied health care providers about MS and to promote the education of patients, their families and the general public about the disease.

Veterans Affairs (VA) MS Centers of Excellence

MSCoE has been established by the US Department of Veterans Affairs to promote the best possible care for veterans with Multiple Sclerosis and provide valuable Multiple Sclerosis resources for VA health care providers. MSCoE "hubs" are located in Baltimore (MSCoE East) and Seattle/Portland (MSCoE West).

East of the Mississippi

Baltimore VA Medical Center
MS Center of Excellence
10 North Green Street
Baltimore, MD 21201
(800) 463-6295
www.vamhcs.med.va.gov/balto/baltimore.htm

West of the Mississippi

VA Puget Sound Health Care System
Seattle Division
MS Center of Excellence
1660 South Columbian Way
Seattle, WA 98108
(206) 762-1010
www.puget-sound.med.va.gov and
http://faculty.washington.edu/hatzakis/COE/Index.html

Portland VA Medical Center
MS Center of Excellence
3710 SW US Veterans Hospital Road
Portland, OR 97239
(503) 220-8262
www.portland.med.va.gov

American Academy of Physical Medicine and Rehabilitation
IBM Plaza, Suite 2500
Chicago, IL 60611-3604
(312) 464-9700
www.aapmr.org

Rehabilitation physicians are nerve, muscle, bone and brain experts who treat injury or illness nonsurgically to decrease pain and restore function. The American Academy of Physical Medicine and Rehabilitation is a national medical society representing more than 7,500 physicians who are specialists in the field of physical medicine and rehabilitation (PM&R).

Caregiving

Family Caregiver Alliance
180 Montgomery Street, Suite 1100
San Francisco, CA 94104
(415) 434-3388
(800) 445-8106
www.caregiver.org

Family Caregiver Alliance (FCA) seeks to improve the quality of life for caregivers through education, services, research and advocacy, offers information on current social, public policy and caregiving issues and provides assistance in the development of public and private programs for caregivers.

For residents of the greater San Francisco Bay Area, FCA provides direct family support services for caregivers of those with

Alzheimer's disease, stroke, MS, ALS, head injury, Parkinson's and other debilitating disorders that strike adults.

National Council on Independent Living
1916 Wilson Blvd, Suite 209
Arlington, VA 22201
(703) 525-3406
www.ncil.org

The National Council on Independent Living is the longest-running national cross-disability, grassroots organization run by and for people with disabilities. Founded in 1982, NCIL represents thousands of organizations and individuals that advocate for the human and civil rights of people with disabilities throughout the United States. NCIL advances independent living and the rights of people with disabilities through consumer-driven advocacy.

Well Spouse Foundation
63 West Main Street, Suite H
Freehold, NJ 07728
(800) 838-0879
www.wellspouse.org

Well Spouse is a national not for profit organization founded in 1988 by author and spousal caregiver, Maggie Strong, whose husband was diagnosed with Multiple Sclerosis (MS). It provides emotional peer-to-peer support to the wives, husbands, and partners of the chronically ill and/or disabled and its members share information on a wide range of practical issues facing spousal caregivers.

MS Friends
2370 Market Street #347
San Francisco, CA 94114
Telephone: (866) 673-7436
www.msfriends.org

MSFriends' mission is to improve the quality of life for people with Multiple Sclerosis and for their families and friends. MSFriends offers a 24/7 telephone helpline staffed with people who have MS that offer MSFriends Guided Outreach to anyone, anywhere.

Lotsa Helping Hands
2 Clock Tower Place, Suite 610
Maynard, MA 01754
http://nac.lotsahelpinghands.com

Lotsa Helping Hands is a private, web-based caregiving coordination service that allows family, friends, neighbors and colleagues to create a community and assist with the daily tasks that become a challenge during long-term caregiving.

Send Us Your Story

Do you have a story to tell? LaChance Publishing and The Healing Project publish four books a year of stories written by people like you. Have you or those you know been touched by life-threatening illness or chronic disease? Your story can give comfort, courage and strength to others who are going through what you have already faced.

Your story should be no less than 500 words and no more than 2,000 words. You can write about yourself or someone you know. Your story must inform, inspire, or teach others. Tell the story of how you or someone you know faced adversity; what you learned that would be important for others to know; how dealing with the disease strengthened or clarified your relationships or inspired positive changes in your life.

The easiest way to submit your story is to visit the LaChance Publishing website at www.lachancepublishing.com. There you will find guidelines for submitting your story online, or you may write to us at submissions@lachancepublishing.com. We look forward to reading your story!